The
Lazy Girl's
Guide to a Fabulous
Body

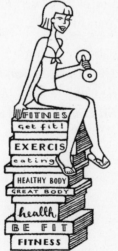

Anita Naik is a freelance writer who has written for *Red*, *New Woman*,
M magazine, *Cosmopolitan*, *Glamour*, *Now* and *Men's Health*.
She specialises in health, beauty, sex and relationships and is currently
the health and advice columnist for *Closer*, and a sex columnist
on *More* magazine.

Anita is also the author of:
The Lazy Girl's Guide to Beauty
The Lazy Girl's Guide to Good Health
The Lazy Girl's Guide to Good Sex

The Lazy Girl's Guide to a Fabulous Body

Anita Naik

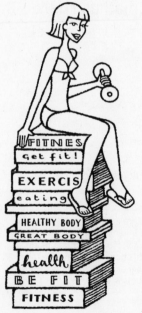

PIATKUS

✿ *Visit the Piatkus website!*

Piatkus publishes a wide range of bestselling fiction and non-fiction, including books on health, mind, body & spirit, sex, self-help, cookery, biography and the paranormal.

If you want to:

- read descriptions of our popular titles
- buy our books over the internet
- take advantage of our special offers
- enter our monthly competition
- learn more about your favourite Piatkus authors

VISIT OUR WEBSITE AT: www.piatkus.co.uk

First published in 2003 by
Judy Piatkus (Publishers) Limited
5 Windmill Street
London W1T 2JA

e-mail: info@piatkus.co.uk

The moral right of the author has been asserted

A catalogue record for this book is available from the British Library

ISBN 0 7499 2432 2

The opinions and advice expressed in this book are intended as a guide only. Neither the publisher nor the author is engaged in rendering professional advice or services to the individual reader. If you have a medical condition or are pregnant, the diet and exercises described in this book should not be followed without first consulting your doctor. The publisher and the author accept no responsibility for any loss or injury as a result of using this book.

Text design by skeisch and Paul Saunders
Edited by Jan Cutler
Cover and inside illustrations by Nicola Cramp
Exercise illustrations by Alison Sturgeon

This book has been printed on paper manufactured with respect for the environment using wood from managed sustainable resources

Printed and bound in Great Britain by Antony Rowe Ltd, Chippenham, Wiltshire

contents

acknowledgements

For all their expert advice and ideas, grateful thanks go to personal trainer Kieran Mullins and Pilates queen Sinéad Harrison. For being fabulously good at 'trying out' the bikini-fit plan much appreciation goes to my favourite lazy girls – Alison Ive, Emma B and Alice Davis at Piatkus Books.

Kieran Mullins is a personal trainer with over ten years of experience in physiology, biomechanics and nutrition. He has a degree in physical education, and YMCA Personal Training and Holmes Place Academy of Personal Trainers qualifications. He's also trained to coach football and boxing, and currently works as trainer for Holmes Place Health Clubs in North London. Kieran is also the owner of OUTFIT – a sportswear shop in London's Crouch End.

Sinéad Harrison has been teaching Pilates for over eight years. She has worked with the Central School of Ballet and is a teacher at Pilates Off the Square in London (www.pilatesoffthesquare.co.uk). She is also a registered teacher with the The Pilates Foundation (www.pilatesfoundation.com).

introduction

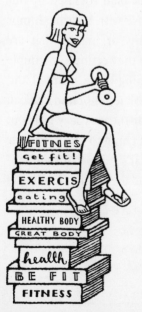

Why this book can help you

If you haven't done a sliver of exercise since you were forced to don PE knickers and go on a run in freezing temperatures, the thought of exercising probably turns your stomach faster than the thought of a stick of celery for lunch. And who could blame you? Exercise is generally divided into those who can (those annoying runner types and the equally irritating bendy yoga girls) and those who can't (er ... probably you). However, while you might laugh at having a stomach that concertinas when you sit down, and scoff at those who don't drink because they're going to the gym at 8.00 a.m., in secret you probably wish you could look better than you do.

The good news is if you're too lazy to move your bottom, but still worried about how it's started to sweep the floor then *The Lazy Girl's Guide to a Fabulous Body* is the perfect book for you. Aimed at those who want to look great but don't want to invest all their spare time in going exercising, this guide can help you to get fit right now. Even better, you can use this book in a variety of ways: to prop your head up while you're watching TV, to show your friends when they bring up the sentence, 'You really should do some exercise', and/or to stop the table from wobbling while you eat your extra-large double-cheese pizza.

Or you can follow it word for word, especially if you're looking for a total body re-haul. The eager (and the serious) can try the bikini-fit six-week plan (devised by our fabulous expert trainer), while those with horrible lumps and bumps, such as batwing arms or breasts that are weighed down by gravity, can try the section on trouble spots (Chapter 5). For those yearning to be sculpted and lean, Chapter 3 (devised by our Pilates supremo) has all the tips you'll ever need. Finally, for the very lazy girls out there who know that they're never going to make it to the end of the book, there is even a cheat's guide to instant fabulousness (ironically, at the end of the book). Try it and thank us later.

chapter 1
Getting psyched

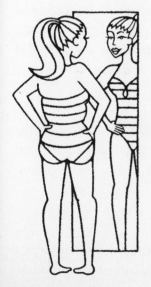

You want to look fabulous and who can blame you? You don't want lazy girl thighs that rub when you walk, underarms that flap in the wind and a sagging cellulite-speckled bottom that screams 'couch potato' when you're on the beach. Well, if you want to look great in a bikini, and have calves that are slim enough to fit into knee-length boots (and knee-fat overlap doesn't count) you've come to the right place. The good news is you can have a fabulous body *and* without going through major surgery and starvation.

However, let's be honest: if you want to get into shape, it's not going to happen if the place you're most likely to be found is on the sofa, and the only exercise you get is walking to the fridge and back. To reach the state of fabulousness (plus get through the whole of this book), here are the rules:

Rule 1: *stop whining about the state of your body*
Constant self-flagellation not only stops you from heaving yourself off the sofa and doing something positive but also will have you reaching for something to eat faster than an advert for chocolate. It also makes you boring, not only to your friends, who are probably sick of telling you you're gorgeous, but also to yourself.

Rule 2: *be honest with yourself*
You don't have to tell anyone else that the reason you're spilling over your jeans is because you eat ten chocolate bars a day, but you do have to admit this to yourself. Otherwise, you're likely to take up all the advice in this book and still spill over your jeans (and then blame us)!

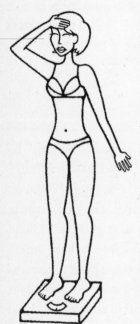

Rule 3: *stop making excuses*
Telling friends you would exercise/lose weight/get healthy BUT … is just another way of saying you can't be bothered to do anything, which is fine, but if you're serious, stop talking and start doing.

Rule 4: *be realistic about your goals*
You may dream of looking like a tiny pop star with a pert bum, but if you're carrying the world behind you, you never

will, unless of course you intend to put in 110 per cent (and if you've bought this book I'm guessing this is not you).

Rule 5: *give yourself a break*

You're human and despite your good intentions there will come a point in your week when you'll want a chocolate brownie loaded with cream, and if you want to eat it, then eat it. However, bear in mind that you should probably eat just one and that points 2 and 3 should then be stapled to your head.

Rule 6: *tell yourself you can do it*

Millions of people transform themselves all the time, and they don't just pile the weight back on, and/or lose their minds in the process. Follow the tips in this book and we guarantee you will feel and look better. Follow them precisely and you'll look fabulous.

tip

Whining about your body won't do anything but bore your friends and make you depressed.

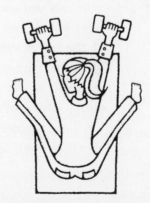

What's holding you back?

Of course, all of us have good intentions when it comes to getting in shape. We all plan that tomorrow/next week/ next month we'll get fit, lose weight, eat healthily and stop drinking our body weight in alcohol. The great majority of us then flunk out big time, simply because our new plans are so alien to the way we actually live our lives, there's no way we're going to fulfil them.

Meaning, no lazy girl is going to get up at 7.00 a.m., eat a healthy breakfast and get into the gym before work. Neither is she going to opt for a salad on her way home from the pub at 11.00 p.m. So, if you're someone who parties hard, has no idea where the kitchen is in your house, and thinks an Egg McMuffin contains all the essential nutrients you need for breakfast, then it's highly unlikely any health regime is going to sit well with you.

Not that this means you're not the healthy type. Studies show that with a bit of determination and effort you can do anything you set your mind to; the emphasis being on firmly setting your mind to it. Therefore, before you do anything, you need to make a plan and jump over the hurdles that are holding you back.

Hurdle one: your beliefs

If you've always been slightly out of shape and/or have no history of being particularly athletic, sporty or healthy (in other words, you were the last one picked for team sports at school) then it's likely that you say one or all of the following to yourself:

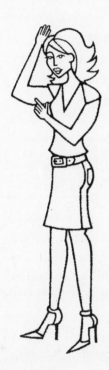

You say: I'm not the sporty type.

We say: Anyone can be sporty, and at any time in their lives. Thankfully childhood PE lessons are not an indication of what you can achieve as an adult.

You say: This is my natural shape.

We say: Doubtful. Give yourself six weeks of exercise and then come back to us.

You say: I can't lose weight.

We say: Oh yes, you can. You may have been on every diet known to man, but studies show the weight loss equation is simple – eat less and do more (and stick to it).

You say: I'm big boned.

We say: It makes no difference what your build is as your weight is a different factor.

myth

'It's not my fault, it's my genes.' Unlikely, only 1 per cent of the population can blame their parents for their weight, and yet 60 per cent of adults are overweight.

Hurdle two: your inner laziness

OK, so the mind's willing but your body's not. Continue to make excuses and you'll continue to be unhappy with the way you look. Popular beliefs on exercising are:

You say: I have no time.

We say: Get up earlier, or forgo your lunch hour, or spend one hour less in the pub or watching TV and you'll suddenly have time to exercise.

You say: I'm too stressed.

We say: All the more reason to eat healthily and do some exercise, as this is known to combat stress instantaneously.

You say: I have no one to exercise with.

We say: Do it yourself (after all you manage to be unhealthy on your own). Better still, inspire some friends to do it with you, join a gym – they're not as expensive as you think – and/or find a local running club.

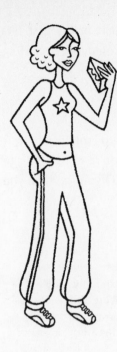

You say: Why fight nature?

We say: You're not fighting nature, you're fighting your habits!

Hurdle three: you don't know where to start

Sometimes trying to change your body and attitude feels as big a challenge as trying to climb Everest. Where to start is actually not as important as actually starting. Whether you've got weight to lose, muscles to firm, and/or eating habits that need to be revised, it's always a case of less thinking and more doing.

You say: What's the point in exercising if I am overweight?

We say: Exercising is not just about pummelling your body into shape. It's about helping you to feel fantastic (it gives you an amazing endorphin release), plus it speeds up your metabolism, meaning you will burn more calories and so see faster results.

You say: I have so much weight to lose it will take me years.

We say: Healthy weight loss occurs at about 900g (2lb) a week; in a month that equals 3.5kg (8lb – over half a stone), which is pretty fast! And if you have a large amount to lose, you'll lose even more than that in the first few weeks. In six months this means you could lose over 19kg (3 stone).

You say: I'll never look the way I want.

We say: It depends on what you want to look like. If your goals are specific and realistic (i.e., you're not hoping to reach supermodel status or run in the Olympics) then you can do it.

myth

If I start dieting and exercising and then stop, my body will look worse. No, lean muscle mass, and fat are different body tissues and so if you stop exercising, you won't turn to jelly because of muscle loss, but because you're eating too much.

Hurdle four: no one thinks you can do it

Most people think they're supportive and encouraging but the fact is most people aren't. If you're someone who has tried and failed numerous times to get fit/lose weight and/or get healthy, it's likely your friends and family either glaze over or laugh hysterically whenever you mention a new plan.

You say: No one thinks I can do it.

We say: Who cares? As long as you think you can do it, you can, as it's your input and belief that is the most important factor in getting fit.

You say: People always put my ideas down.

We say: All new ideas are easily squashed, which is why it's important to pick the right people to support your new-found enthusiasm. Avoid those who can't wait to tell you why it won't work, why it will go wrong and why you won't do it. Instead choose someone who's already been there and done it.

tip

You'll never reach your destination if you don't know where you're going. This means it's no use being vague about what being fabulous means – figure out your definition and stick to it.

You say: I can't find the right support.

We say: Sometimes, as much as we love our friends and family, they aren't our best cheerleaders. If the right support is not around, go out and find it. Think about a personal trainer, a slimming group, or even a local running group. Better still, join a fitness class and make new friends with people who have similar goals to you.

You say: My boyfriend keeps trying to sabotage my efforts.

We say: He's feeling insecure. Maybe he thinks you're going to get a fabulous body and run off – reassure him this isn't the case, but be firm about what you're doing and what you need from him.

Create your own lazy girl goals

Saying you want to look better than you do right now, get to a healthy weight and have more energy are all worthy goals, but they're not very inspiring, or motivating, which means they won't get you through your darkest hours. So let's be shallow about it. Aim for something that you'd maybe only confess to your best friend: perhaps to be able to get into a thong bikini or a sexy little black dress. Or maybe to make your ex sorry he left, or to get the kind of body that makes people look twice at you when you walk into a room.

Goal 1: inspire yourself

Think about what would inspire you to keep going when all you want to do is lie on the sofa and eat crisps because it is this that will motivate you to change your habits.

Goal 2: write your plan down

The process of making your goals happen occurs when you start to make it real. Whether you choose to make your goals public or not, you have to be able to see what you're aiming for every day. So arm yourself with a notebook and write down what you want to achieve (it doesn't matter what it is, this is for your eyes only) and review it regularly.

Goal 3: pick a short-term goal

This is essential because if you don't reap some rewards for your hard work in the short term, you'll give up in the long term. Every four weeks make a new short-term goal to move you forwards.

Goal 4: choose a long-term goal

This is the goal that usually stays the same. However, you may find that what you originally set out to do becomes less important as you get near to it (or you'll find that what you're really aiming for is something else entirely), either way it doesn't really matter.

Goal 5: be wary of the reward system

Lots of fitness experts and coaches, advocate treating yourself when you do something you hate, such as exercising or losing weight. The danger with this, however, is you train your mind to think that exercise/healthy eating and a change of attitude is a horrible thing, when in fact it's easier and less painful than you think (the main part of the pain is making yourself do it).

Goal 6: get your head round what you can and can't do

This is another 'be realistic' point. If you are pushed for time or like your morning lie-ins, then don't aim to exercise at 7.0 a.m. in the morning because you'll do it for a

tip

Short-term goals can be anything from making yourself join a gym and getting a personal trainer to drinking fewer than 14 units of alcohol a week. Or it could be something more specific, such as losing 2.25kg (5lb) by the end of the month.

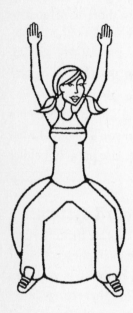

week and then give up. Likewise, if you eat at home only one day a week, don't aim to follow a specific and rigid diet that you have no hope of maintaining in Burger King.

Goal 7: don't be an 'if only ...' person

Make your plan work with some forward thinking. If you travel a lot for work, ensure you follow your plan on days that you're home, and work out a way to do it when you're away (see Chapter 6). If you are on a shift-work pattern, exercise on your free days and plan your meals. Finally, think about the weekend. Just because these are your free days doesn't mean, you can't follow your plan then as well. Remember your goals are for every day, not just for the days when you can be bothered.

Find your lazy girl willpower

When it comes to willpower more of us score a big fat zero. Funny then that we can get out of bed at 5.0 a.m. to catch a plane to go on holiday, stay up dancing until 3.0 a.m. and then still be at work for 9.0 a.m.! Amazing then that we can say no to a second piece of chocolate cake because a good-looking waiter is serving us, or eat nothing all day because we want to get trashed at night.

If this shows anything, it's that if you put your mind to it you can do anything.

If you don't believe me, think of a time when you aimed for something wonderful and succeeded. Maybe you landed a job you really wanted, asked a man out you fancied, lost weight for an event, or even passed your driving test. Now consider how you did it, because that technique would pretty much work for anything. Ask yourself:

- What motivated you to achieve this goal?
- How did you keep going when you wanted to give up?
- Who (or what) did you get to help you, and why?
- What could you use from this experience to motivate you to get fabulous?

If you have thought about taking your driving test, it's likely that the thought of owning your own car motivated you to pass your test (your goal). The horrible idea that you'd have to rely on your parents and friends for lifts kept you going when lessons got hard (your motivation), and a parent or a driving instructor (i.e., an expert) helped teach you the things you needed to know in order to pass.

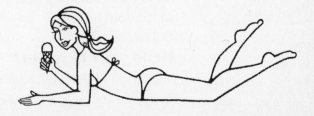

> ## To achieve any goal you need the following:
>
> - To know the benefits you'd personally reap if you achieved your aim.
> - What would happen to you if you didn't; i.e., how bad you'd be feeling a year from now.
> - Advice and support from an expert to help point you in the right direction.

Not convinced this technique would work in this area? Then find someone who has reached the goal you're trying to get to, and talk to him or her about how they did it. All of us have a recipe for success even if we don't know what it is. This means, if you can discover someone else's pattern, you can amend it and make it work for you. For example, if your aim is to lose weight, ask someone who has achieved fantastic results how he or she did it (use the four questions above). This way you'll discover tips they used to motivate themselves, techniques they followed to boost their willpower and patterns you can follow to achieve your own goal.

Move your lazy butt

OK, so you've thought about it, mulled it over, written a list, a plan and told all your best friends. Now it's time to

Good motivators

- A deadline.
- Best friends.
- Keeping a cut-out picture of the ideal bikini/jeans you want to wear.
- A tape measure – measuring by centimetre (inch) loss is more satisfying than going by kilograms (pounds) lost.
- Having a picture of you looking super-sexy – something to better and maintain.
- A photograph of you looking not so good – something to remind you why you're doing this.

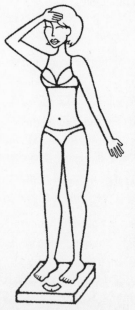

Bad motivators

- Buying new clothes two sizes smaller.
- Telling everyone you are dieting and going to the gym.
- Asking your boyfriend to berate you every time you eat chocolate.
- A picture of a celebrity.
- Bathroom scales.
- A fat picture of you on the fridge (guaranteed to have you reaching for another biscuit).

take action. If you're telling yourself you're going to start in the summer because it's easier to get up early then, or when you get a raise because then you can afford a trainer, or in a few weeks' time when you're feeling up to it – you're lying to yourself. If you're serious about getting started take action right now.

Things you can take immediate action on

- Ditching all the junk food in your fridge. If it's in the bin you can't eat it.
- Looking up the number of your nearest gym/swimming pool/yoga class and calling them for a timetable.
- Buying a workout video.
- Finding your Nikes.
- Making a meal that's low fat instead of opting for a takeaway.
- Snacking on fruit.
- Doing five press-ups right now on the floor.
- Taking a long, but fast-paced, walk to a café and reading the rest of this chapter there.

How to take action is simple

1. Firstly, pick a date. If you're really not ready today, pick one somewhere in the next week and then don't put off that date for anything. Not for bad weather, a night out or stress at work.
2. Next, buy yourself something for this event (remember this is the start of the new fabulous YOU). Workout gear, new trainers and even a blank book where you can chart your progress.

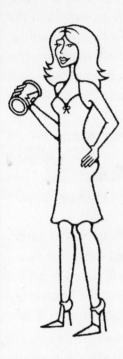

3. Now prepare for the start. If your aim is to change your diet, make sure your cupboards are clear of anything you may be tempted by. Either have a blow-out party, and load it all on your friends, or ditch it in the bin and make sure you dump it outside. Now fill your kitchen in advance with the things you hope to be eating. If your plan is to exercise, make sure you have your workout gear ready to go the day before. If it's packed you'll have no excuse to avoid the inevitable.

4. Ask one friend to call you up and encourage you (just one, otherwise the pressure will be too much) and if you can get this person to come along with you all the better. However, be careful who you choose as your fabulous buddy, try to pick someone who will inspire you, not back up your excuses. The perfect buddy is someone who genuinely wants you to succeed, or, has once been in the same place herself, and so can offer you helpful advice.

5. Finally, ignore those who have nothing helpful to offer. Life is full of people who want to stop you from doing what they can't be bothered to do. Hints that you're facing such a person include someone who tells you that exercise is a waste of time, that dieting doesn't work, and that you're getting a bit obsessive about your plans.

Make it a habit

For most of us the hardest part of any fitness/diet/health plan is to take it from the idea stage to the doing stage. How many times have you lounged about in your workout gear telling yourself 'I must get to the gym' only to find three hours have passed and you're still on the sofa? If this sounds like you, then you need to realise that commitment is something you have to build in yourself, something that grows with repetition and results, i.e., the more you do it and the more results you see the more committed you become.

To beat the 'I can't be bothered today' feeling, make a timetable that you can't avoid with excuses. Fix an exact time to workout every day so it isn't a vague idea. Then choose a place near your workplace, or a place you actually have to pass to get home.

If you're planning to eat healthily, change where you eat and shop so you won't be tempted by old habits. For example, don't go out for lunch at the café where you have previously ordered chips and a sandwich for lunch every day. Either pick a new place where you can start a new habit or bring your lunch in.

Do it even when it's difficult. This is especially important in the early days. If you give yourself an excuse because you feel tired/stressed or because it's the weekend you'll find one for tomorrow and the one after and the one after that!

Start as soon as possible. Ideas wither if you keep them hanging around. To become the fabulous person you want to be – start ASAP … and don't procrastinate.

20 get-psyched lazy tips

1 Take action right now
It takes two weeks to replace a habit with a new behaviour, and six to nine weeks to then make this feel like second nature. Put your plan into action now and you'll be a new woman sooner than you think!

2 Pick the right team-mates
As much as you love all your friends and family, they won't all be on your side. Some will feel threatened by your new-found zest for health, some will think you're bonkers and others will willingly try to sabotage your efforts. Be aware of what's happening around you. Choose the right team-mates.

3 Think of the future
If your willpower is flagging, imagine how you'd feel a year from now if you were still in the same place. Picture yourself, and then every time you feel you can't be bothered to stick to your plan, conjure up that image.

4 Preparation is the key
Those cub scouts had it right – be prepared and you can do anything. This means prepare for the new you. If you're a fly-by-the-seat-of-your-pants kind of girl, you'll never create a new habit.

5 Be proud of what you're doing
Most of us find getting fit and losing weight embarrassing, as if it's a public confession to everyone that we have horrible flaws. The fact is you should hold your head up proudly if you're doing something, because 75 per cent of people do nothing at all.

6 Ask for help
Never be afraid to ask for someone's help when you're trying to achieve something. Those who ask – get! Speak to people in health-food shops, someone who has lost loads of weight and/or that scary girl at the gym who runs at 100 mph. You never know what tips you'll get.

7 All it takes is one decision to change your life

If you want to lose weight, tone your thighs, firm your batwing arms, get more energy, improve your skin ... all it takes is a decision to start doing some exercise that will get you on the road to wherever you want to go.

8 Persist when things get hard

Easier said than done, but making your plan work on the days when it's horribly hard will give you a huge sense of achievement and stop self-flagellation in its tracks.

9 Work harder when it gets easy

It sounds weird, but when things get easy that's the sign that you need to hike things up a level because your body and mind have got too used to it. Whether this means rewriting a goal, running faster or changing your diet only you can say.

10 Give yourself a new label

Ever had someone say to you, 'Oh I can't imagine YOU doing that ...' well, apart from hitting them over the head, this is a sign that you need to give yourself a new label. Tell yourself you're an exerciser, healthy eater, whatever it is you're aiming at. This will reinforce the idea that you're doing it, living it and being it.

11 Information is power

The more you know, the more you'll do. Whatever your goal – read up on it. You don't have to immerse yourself in the boring stuff, but start reading relevant magazines and watching programmes that are geared in that direction; it will cement the idea in your head.

12 Don't kick yourself when you're down

We all have bad days – don't use this as an excuse to throw in the towel and give up. Just because you've fallen off track doesn't mean you can't just jump back on tomorrow.

13 Give yourself a deadline

Plans that have no fixed deadline

tend to wobble and fall. It's a bit like promising yourself you'll give up smoking tomorrow. The problem is tomorrow literally never comes. Which is why with health and fitness goals you need to choose a focal point to move towards.

14 Check what you say to yourself

Look at the ways you hinder yourself. Do you often tell yourself that you can't do something/won't be able to do it/that you're lazy and meant to be fat? If so, these are not truths, but self-sabotaging techniques (you probably use them in other areas of your life as well) that you've said so often that you don't think twice about them.

15 Don't overdo it

While enthusiasm is great, be wary of burning yourself out too fast. The aim is to work at a steady pace, not go at 100 mph for three weeks and then retire to the sofa with a packet of Pringles. Find the pace that is right for you and you'll stick to it.

16 Don't let people bully you

OK, so you asked for support but this doesn't mean you should allow 'friends' to bully you, and comment on everything that goes into your mouth. You know what you have to do and how to get there (or you will by the end of this book) so don't let others be your conscience.

17 See possibilities in your plan

Aside from what you'll eventually achieve, think about what you're going to get out of your plan on a daily basis. If fitness is your goal, tell yourself you'll be able to do things that you once thought were out of your reach – go on a hike, climb a mountain (well a big hill), have sex for longer, even run a marathon!

18 Add up all the pluses

So your goal is to get into a size ten pair of jeans, but what about all the other pluses that your plan will give you? Think less stress, better sleep, fantastic skin, more confidence, happier moods, and, above all, better self-esteem.

19 Break your goals into small chunks

Feeling that you can't do it? Well no matter how huge and vast your goal you can do it if you break it into small manageable pieces (just the way you once managed to eat your way through a family bar of chocolate). You're not going to do something overnight but you can make a start overnight.

20 Feel pleased with yourself

Go on, give yourself a congratulatory pat on the back. Apart from the fact you've reached the end of Chapter 1, you're already doing more for your body than the great majority of people out there.

chapter 2
The lazy girl food rules

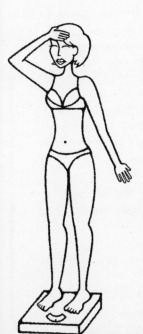

Hands up if you know what healthy eating is? If the words fruit, vegetables and 'foods I don't eat' all fall into your answer, then this is the chapter for you. Contrary to popular belief healthy eating is not just about losing weight and becoming a size ten but also about feeling good and looking good. Thankfully it's not about forbidding yourself all the food you like and eating lettuce leaves and cottage cheese for every meal. It's not even about detoxing or cutting out entire food groups.

Healthy eating is about having a healthy attitude to food. Eating when you're hungry, choosing foods that give you energy and vitamins, and not beating yourself over the head when you have a blow out and eat chocolate cake all day. It sounds simple enough and yet most of us, if we're honest, have a more than tricky relationship with food and how much we do or don't eat.

If you want to lose weight, the equation is simple and not rocket science: eat less and do more and you'll lose the excess pounds. You might think (or hope) it's more complicated than that so you can have an excuse to do nothing about it, but that's the truth. Your genes only make up a small part of the equation, as does your build, which means at the end of the day it's all down to what you choose to put into your mouth. Regularly scoff takeaways, crisps, chocolates and biscuits and you're going to gain

Healthy eating is ...

- Eating a variety of foods with every meal.
- Having three meals a day and two snacks.
- Eating food for energy, vitamins and nutrients as well as pleasure.
- Eating vegetables and fruit daily.
- Eating every four hours so you never feel starving.
- Listening to your hunger signals before you eat.
- Not being obsessive about what you eat.
- Being honest about what you do eat.
- Admitting that there are just some things you can't have if you're trying to lose weight.
- Drinking at least 1.5 litres of water a day.
- Cutting back on drinks high in sugar.

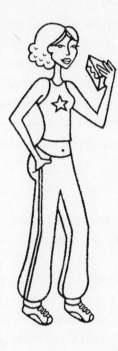

weight. Do no exercise, snack constantly and choose meals that you know have a high fat and calorie content and your belly will remain wobbly for life. The good news is it's easy to adopt a healthy-eating strategy that will help you lose weight, feel healthier and look better. It won't cost you an arm and a leg, your social life, or even your daily bar of chocolate.

Healthy eating isn't ...

- Having just a coffee for breakfast.
- Skipping breakfast (or any other meal) entirely.
- Cutting out entire food groups.
- Eating boring foods.
- Dieting/losing weight and then going back to your 'normal' way of eating.
- Taking diet pills.
- Refusing to eat at other people's houses because you're worried about your diet.
- Opting for a Mars bar rather than a sandwich.
- Being obsessive about wheat and dairy.
- Telling people you don't have time to eat properly.
- Starving yourself one day and over-compensating the next.

What's your weight?

Why be thinner? Why indeed? The truth is you don't have to lose weight or be thinner if you don't want to. Nobody is forcing you to diet (unless your weight is affecting your health, in which case it pays to listen to your doctor). However, if you're reading this book then I'd say a part of you, no matter how small, wants to lose a few pounds or more. To work out if you really are overweight take a look at the following methods:

1 Body mass index (BMI)

This is a scale now used by all health professionals to assess your weight in relation to your height and tells you how healthy your current shape is.

To find your BMI, all you have to do is divide your weight in kilos (1lb = 0.45kg, and there are 14lb in a stone) by your height in metres squared (1ft = 30.48cm).

So if you weigh 10 stone, that's 140lbs × 0.45kg = 63kg

If youre 5ft 6in, that's 5.6 × 30.48cm = 1. 70m

To square your height, 1.70 × 1.70 = 2.89

Then divide your weight, 63kg, by your height, 2.89 = a BMI of 22

- A BMI of 20 is considered underweight.
- A BMI of 20–24 is considered normal.
- A BMI of over 25 to less than 30 is considered overweight.
- A BMI of over 30 is considered obese.

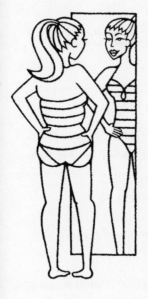

2 Scale weight

Measuring your weight on scales only reflects how weight changes for you. This means that unless you measure your reading against an official standard, such as a chart, you cannot assess your weight/health risk and level of body fatness. Plus, weight loss seen on scales sometimes reflects fluid loss, rather than actual fat loss, which is deceiving, plus it fluctuates at different times of the month.

3 Body-fat percentage tests

This is difficult to do accurately, but it can be done at a gym or larger chemists and has the advantage of giving an indication of fatness. Remember that as a woman you will always have a higher body-fat percentage than a man will. A healthy range for women is between 18–28 per cent (for men it's between 12–18 per cent). Though remember you do not have to be overweight to be over-fat. Do zero exercise and your body will have little lean muscle mass and a lot of fat.

4 Waist circumference

This test has the advantage of assessing the level (but not amount) of excess abdominal/central weight you have. It's this weight that carries the greatest risk for health problems such as diabetes, heart disease and high blood pressure. For men, a waist measurement of 94–102cm (37–40in) means 'alert' (either don't gain weight or lose some weight), while 102cm (40in) or more means 'red alert' (obesity). For women it's 81–89cm (32–35in) and 89cm (35in) or more, respectively. To measure your waist, make sure the tape goes around the belly-button area.

Common myths about weight loss

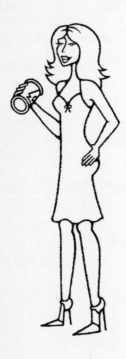

Myth: *some people are just meant to be fat.*

Truth: you can be any size and weight you choose to be. If that wasn't true obese people would never be able to lose 63.5kg (140lb, or 10 stone), slim people wouldn't gain weight, and exercise would be a waste of time.

Myth: *don't eat after 7.00 p.m., as all the calories are then stored as fat.*

Truth: this is a pure piece of nonsense. It's not when you eat but how much you eat overall that affects your fat levels. People who eat after 7.00 p.m. burn exactly the same calories as those who eat their main meal at lunch.

Myth: *you can work off that piece of cake.*

Truth: you can, but its hard, hard work. One piece of cake will take half an hour to run off.

myth

Calories from fat make you gain weight faster than calories from carbohydrates. No, the truth is that excess calories from anything make you gain weight.

Myth: *I have a slow metabolism so I'll never lose weight.*

Truth: even the slowest of metabolisms will burn fat when faced with a programme of healthy eating and exercise. To raise your metabolism you have to work to increase lean muscle tissue (done by building muscle, see Chapter 5).

Myth: *size is hereditary.*

Truth: only 1 per cent of the population can blame their parents, currently 40 per cent of the UK population and 60 per cent of the US population are overweight.

Myth: *to lose weight you need to cut carbohydrates.*

Truth: the opposite – you need to increase your carbohydrates because they're better for your overall health and have fewer calories than fat products.

Myth: *you can eat as much as you want if it's fat-free or low fat.*

Truth: fat-free doesn't mean calorie-free or sugar-free, and low fat doesn't mean low calorie, so both will still help you to gain weight.

Myth: *you can diet without doing any exercise.*

Truth: you can but you'll do it quicker if you boost your metabolic rate through exercise.

Myth: *a vegetarian diet is less fattening.*

Truth: many vegetarians eat too much fat, such as cheese (it gives their food flavour), and don't eat enough vegetables. They also often load up on pasta and bread, which are high in calories, making their diet just as unhealthy.

Myth: *eating breakfast makes you hungrier.*

Truth: eating breakfast kick-starts your metabolism, and though you are hungry by lunch this is good news because it means you have been burning calories all morning and need food for energy, not just because it's lunchtime.

Eat well and you'll feel ...

Sexier

Notice I said, 'feel' rather than 'will be'. Sexiness is a state of mind, and if your mind is telling you it's happy with your body then you're going to feel and act sexy no matter what

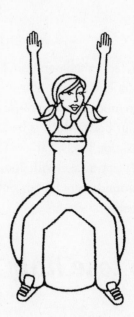

your weight. If, however, you're afraid of taking your clothes off with the lights on, or are too busy sucking in your stomach to have a good roll between the sheets, then you need to boost your self-esteem. The quickest way to do this is to get to grips with your body. You don't have to lose weight to tone up, and you don't have to tone up to lose weight, though obviously both work very well together. Pick an area of your body you'd like to work on, and attach a realistic eating or exercise goal to it (i.e., a goal you know you'll happily stick with).

Energetic

Fresh vegetables, less fat and sugar and more protein means a lighter attitude all round. Not only will such a diet eventually make itself known to your body but also to your mood. Heavily refined foods (processed meals, pasta, sandwiches made with white bread and junk) turn to sugar more quickly in the body, leading to very high and very low blood-sugar levels. This in turn sucks away all the excess energy in the body making you feel sluggish and tired. If you crave sweet stuff and can't get enough of it, stick to fruit (high in natural sugar) or a good dark chocolate, don't give in to coffee and a cake.

Happier

Food is a drug, as it affects your body and brain. Too much sugar, for example, can give you the high followed by a low, explained above. Too much coffee can lead to anxiety and irritability and not enough protein can lead to fatigue. If you want to feel happier, eat properly and more frequently. Choose fresh, raw vegetables, fruit, water, less sugar-based foods and eat every three to four hours to keep your energy up.

More relaxed

The fastest way to stress yourself out, feel irritable and generally angst-ridden is to eat badly. Mood foods (see above) and moods caused by a lack of or too much food can cause your hormones to go haywire in your body, which is bad news for your stress, sleep and relaxation levels. Eat cleverly and wisely and you won't be kept awake with too much caffeine and sugar racing around your blood, or lulled into sleep by a sluggish metabolism.

The only way to lose half a stone is ...

To do it slowly. If the word 'slowly', is putting you off, think again. Three kilograms, or half a stone, is 7lb, which means you can lose it in a month at 450–900g (1–2lb) a week. Lose it any faster and you're not losing fat but water and lean tissue mass (the stuff you need to burn off calories faster). Fast weight loss is bad news because it piles back on in no time. To lose it at a steady rate:

- Take responsibility for your eating. Work out your weak times and think of ways to combat your urge to overeat or snack on the wrong foods.
- Ideally make sure your diet is made up of 50 per cent carbohydrates (vegetables, fruit and unrefined carbs, like brown rice and wholemeal bread), 25 per cent protein (lean meats, fish and eggs) and 25 per cent unsaturated fats (nuts, seeds and oily fish).
- Make small changes immediately. Everything counts, so anything you cut out will count too. One less chocolate bar, one less glass of alcohol, fruit instead of chocolate etc. A plain white coffee rather than a latte – that's 150 calories less a day, 1,050 less calories a week.
- Ditch the junk in your cupboards. That's processed foods like white bread, biscuits, crisps, ready-made meals (high in fat and salt) and foods you may be tempted by when you're having a bad day.
- Do some regular exercise. For average base fitness, that's at least 30 minutes a day that leaves you feeling relatively out of breath. To get in shape, lose the wobble and burn fat you have to do more (see Chapters 3, 4 and 6).
- Get active. Walk up stairs, keep the phone in another room so you have to run for it. Shop by foot and carry the shopping

home. It will help build up lean muscle, which is more metabolically active than fat tissue and so burns more calories.

- Watch how you cook your food. Olive oil is good for you, but its still oil, so don't load your pasta with it. Likewise, watch your salad dressings, mayonnaise and how you choose to cook your vegetables (boil or grill, don't fry), as all these work against weight loss.

- Eat your greens and your fruit, for that matter. An apple has 75 calories and a 25g (1oz) chocolate bar 180, which makes the fruit the better option for a faster weight loss.

- Up your water intake. This will help keep you hydrated and you won't mistake your thirst receptors for hunger signals. Drinking a glass of water before you eat also helps you to eat less at mealtimes.

- Finally, eat slowly to help your brain work out if it's eaten enough. Eat on the run and your stomach will be 20 minutes behind your mouth, telling you you're hungry while food is already on the way.

myth

Weight-loss pills are the answer to losing weight. For those waiting for the perfect anti-fat pill, with no side effects – your wait is in vain, as there will never be a pill that will allow you to eat what you want and still keep you thin.

What to avoid in the dieting game

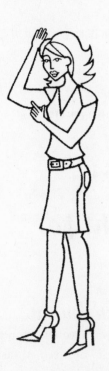

Most countries currently spend in excess of £2 billion a year on diet products. In the US this figure is £45 billion, a fifth of which is spent on products which are totally useless and won't help you lose anything but your patience. Still, the desire to rid ourselves of agonised trips to the bathroom scales means most of us would consider any diet product sold as a sure thing. With even the simplest diets requiring some form of willpower, it isn't hard to understand why we're all seduced by the idea of a miraculous diet or dieter's aid that we can use to lose our excess weight. Eat too much and you'll gain weight; reduce your intake and you'll lose weight. How you choose to do this is up to you, but diets to avoid at all costs include:

- Diets that promise you can lose a large amount of weight in two weeks.
- Diets that all the usual suspects follow (celebrities in particular).
- Diets with a theory that sounds ridiculous.
- Diets that suggest you eat only one thing for a two-week period.
- Diets that suggest you pay X amount for a pill that has a special magic ingredient.

- Diets that mean you have to stay locked in your flat for weeks on end.
- Diets that are totally impractical.
- Diets that say you can eat everything in any amount (sorry but that just doesn't work).
- Diets that cost money to do.
- Diets that have come back in fashion again (they went out of fashion for a reason).
- Diets that mean you have to take pills.
- Diets that make you feel as if you are starving.
- Diets that leave you feeling exhausted (a sign you aren't fuelling your body).
- Diets that doctors say are rubbish.
- Diets that make you fill up on fluids not food.

How to lose weight for good

1 Be honest about how much you eat

If you feel you don't eat much and yet have still gained weight (or haven't lost anything), then you need to take more notice of what goes into your mouth. That's every bite, every snack, every piece of food while you're cooking and every drink, as it all counts. Keep a food diary for three days – you'll be surprised at how much you're really eating.

2 Stop going on mad diets

If your bookshelf is full of every diet book known to man, and you can recite who's been on the eat-no-carbohydrate-drink-watercress-soup-and-eat-like-a-caveman diet then you're a diet junkie and need to go into diet rehab. Firstly, toss away all those useless books, and make a promise to yourself that you won't ever be tempted by a ridiculous diet again. Think sensibly. For all the time and money you have ploughed into your diet-book fixation you could have incorporated healthy-eating tactics, lost weight and saved yourself a ton of money.

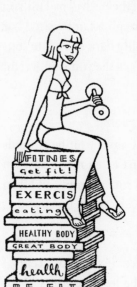

3 Don't compare yourself to others

This is the kiss of death to a good body image. If you're always looking at pictures of celebrities, and negatively comparing yourself to them, it's worth noting a few home truths. Firstly, most celebrities work and diet excessively to get the bodies you see in magazines. For most of them this means 5.00 a.m. runs, evil personal trainers, a rigid diet and no pudding. If you want their body you can get it, but do you really want to go through their regime?

4 Eat like a real person

Eat three meals a day – most people do. It's only mad dieters or deluded women who think that they should only eat one proper meal a day. If you want your metabolism to function properly, eat wisely.

5 Eat a little bit of what you like

Apart from the fact that denying yourself something you want just makes you think about it all the more, naughty delights, such as chocolate, aren't in themselves bad for you (unless of course you're going through a family-sized bar every day). For example, good-quality dark chocolate contains beneficial nutrients and won't make you gain weight unless you eat too much of it.

6 Eat breakfast every day

The reason behind this thinking is simple: your body needs fuel in the morning because it hasn't eaten for at least ten hours. Deprive it of food and it will run on empty and then retaliate at 11.00 a.m. and lunchtime, and pretty much all day.

7 Make fat your friend

If you restrict your fat intake to less than 20 per cent of your calories, studies show you'll be less likely to stick to your diet. Better to go for moderate low-fat food and choose your fats wisely. Unsaturated fats found in oily fish, nuts and seeds and monounsaturated fats found in avocados and olive oil are healthy choices and good for your mood; use them but keep your intake to below 30 per cent.

8 Eat more protein

About 25 per cent of your daily food intake should come from protein because it's essential for building bones,

tip

If you can't be bothered to pour out a bowl of cereal, prepare what you want for breakfast the night before, set your alarm 15 minutes earlier and at least drink a glass of juice before you walk out of the door.

healthy teeth, hair and nails. The best sources are chicken, fish, soya products, milk and eggs. A diet rich in protein (as opposed to protein only) will also control your appetite and stimulate the hormone glucagon to burn fat in the body.

9 Don't be too generous with your servings

Recommended daily servings (RDA) should be: six portions of grains (bread and cereal), five to seven portions of fruit and vegetables, two to three of dairy and two to three of protein.

A serving is smaller than you think

- A medium-sized apple = one serving
- Medium glass of fruit juice = one serving
- Half a cup of cooked vegetables = one serving (so a normal dinner portion of runner beans is already two servings)
- Medium baked potato = one serving
- A medium bagel = two to three servings
- Two to three tablespoons of pasta = one serving
- Small pot of yoghurt = one serving
- Normal glass of milk = one serving

10 Don't overdo it on the fruit front

Some fruits are very high in sugar and calories – so avoid too much pineapple, banana, mango and passion fruit if you want to lose weight. Instead stick to hard fruits and perennials, such as apples. If you're a fan of smoothies, watch how many servings you're having at once and what you're mixing the fruit with (go for skimmed milk or soya milk).

11 Drink more water

Research shows that one in five of us consume too little water throughout the day, bad news when the current recommendation is 1.5 litres (2½ pints), or about eight to ten glasses. Not drinking this means most of us suffer from borderline dehydration every day, which equals tiredness and a tendency to snack for energy. Water is also vital for our optimum health. Not only does it hydrate organs and cushion the nervous system but it also stops you reaching for food when what you really want is a drink (thirst receptors often get mixed up with hunger receptors). Unsure if you need more water? Then look at your urine. The darker the colour the more dehydrated you are, and the more water you need to drink. If the thought of guzzling ten glasses a day is too much for you, think of it as half a glass of water every half an hour, and you'll easily hit your quota.

How much do you want to lose?

If you want to lose 2.25kg (5lb)

Drink more water. Five pounds could be fluid that your body is holding on to because you're dehydrated. Check the colour of your urine: if it's dark you need to drink more.

Cut back on your excesses. This means for a short period cutting out all your faves – sugar, alcohol, refined foods, and ready meals.

Cut out 250 calories a day (the equivalent of two beers or a chocolate bar) you can lose ½lb a week or more. Add more activity to your life. Join an exercise class, run up the stairs at work and add one more gym session a week.

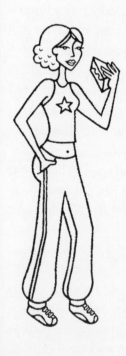

If you want to lose 4.5—7kg (10—15lb)

Step up your intake of fruit and vegetables. You should be looking at five portions (cup size/handful) a day at least. Experts say this is the food group most missing for women who want to lose 4.5kg (10lb).

Make your own meals. This way you can control fat content, portion size and how much you eat at one sitting. It's dull but you have to do it for only a month or two.

Whack up your exercise levels. Running with ease? Then

you need to make your workout more challenging (see Chapters 5 and 6), and start doing free weights to boost your metabolism.

Make one big change. Cut out alcohol, ditch the chocolate or avoid takeaways until you reach your target weight.

If you want to lose 12.75kg (28lb, or 2 stone)

Always see a doctor or dietician (clinically trained nutritionist) first, as you need the right kind of advice and support as to what kind of exercise you should be doing and what kind of diet you should put yourself on. Don't attempt to diet, take up exercise and build up your willpower in one week. Set small goals and make one new change a week. Start by changing your diet, then adding exercise to the equation.

Don't focus on the scales, instead go by how your clothes feel, and set up small goals that you can reach every few weeks. Think about why you eat – it will help boost your willpower.

If you want to de-bloat

For a flat stomach it's essential you avoid eating too many starchy carbohydrates – potatoes, rice, bread and pasta. This is because simple carbohydrates are stored mostly as fat so if you want to stay lean and mean stick to salads, vegetables, chicken and fish.

Don't multi-task and eat. If you eat too fast, or when you're stressed you won't chew food properly, and you'll end up washing your food down and swallowing too much air, which causes stomach bloating, wind and that tight waistband feeling.

Add variety to all your meals. Too many of us eat a diet heavy in wheat – cereals, sandwiches and pasta every day causes bloating and wind problems. Avoid all fizzy canned drinks (diet drinks too), as carbonated drinks lead to bloating. Plus, fizzy drinks of the non-diet variety are packed with sugar. This will not only pile on extra calories but also upset the bacterial balance in your stomach and cause bloating. Also avoid pre-packed processed meals as they are loaded with chemicals, salt and sugar – all things that cause belly bloating and work against flat stomachs.

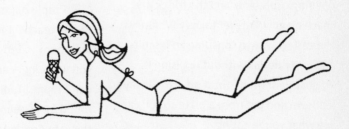

20 lazy diet tips

1 Bite it then write it

Most people don't think they eat that much, simply because they don't count their daily snacking, nibbles and sneaky bites. If you record how much you eat in a three-day period it can be a wake-up call to just how much you're scoffing and will help you to keep your food intake at levels you need, rather than levels you want.

2 Avoid mindless munching

Walking around your kitchen casually opening cupboards and the fridge and snacking on whatever takes your fancy is the easiest way to consume 20 biscuits and 300 calories without realising it. Practise your mum's best advice – always sit down and eat from a plate so you can see what you're eating.

3 Join the breakfast club

Avoid breakfast and by 11.00 a.m. you'll have a hunger attack and eat some-thing that is higher in fat and sugar than a good hearty breakfast. Studies also show that skipping breakfast often leads people to eat more calories per day, as they opt for a larger lunch and more after-noon snacks. If you don't feel hungry first thing, retrain your stomach by slowly introducing food when you get up in the morning. Start with fruit juice, then add cereal – a recent study showed you could lose up to 2.25kg (5lb) in two weeks if you eat cereal twice a day, and then add a daily snack and a normal dinner to the mix.

4 Count to ten before you snack

Simple but effective, say the experts. Before reaching for more, or simply snack-ing, count to ten and think about whether you are hungry and whether you really do want more. Studies by Weight Watchers found most people who counted before they ate decided they really had had enough.

5 Be prepared

The fastest way to eat a Mars bar and

a takeaway pizza five times a week for dinner is to have no easily made food in your house. To combat this always make sure you have food in your fridge or cupboards that takes no more than ten minutes to magic into a meal (and we're not talking ready meals – see above).

6 Don't drink your calories

High-calorie drink choices can sabotage any fitness regime. Aside from alcohol, which is high in calories, think about your mixers. Fruit juices may be good for you but are high in calories (especially if you're having seven helpings in seven vodkas). Coffee is another hidden area. Lattes are crammed full of full-fat milk – opt for a skinny latte or a white coffee. Oversized cream-topped, caramel-coffee concoctions can also add an extra 350 calories to your daily diet.

7 Rethink your portions

Eating wisely but still not losing weight? Well you could be consuming bigger meals than you need. A serving is a handful, meaning a palm-sized piece of chicken or fish for your main meal. Vegetables can be unlimited unless they are fried and coated in butter, in which case be careful. As for fruit, it is good for you but not in large amounts (it's high in sugar), so stick to two servings a day (one apple = one serving).

8 Say no to king-size packs

Studies show that chocolate bars and crisp bags are getting bigger, which is bad news for our thighs. The solution – never buy king-size or family packs because you'll only end up scoffing the lot. Fun-size portions also only work if you have huge amounts of willpower. Stick to a normal bar, especially at the cinema where we're all guilty of eating our way through a family-sized bag of Maltesers or a vat of popcorn (if you wouldn't do it in front of the TV, don't do it at the cinema).

9 Shop when you're full

It's a guaranteed way to avoid filling your trolley with products that would be best suited to a ten-year-old's birthday party. Shopping on empty makes it especially hard to avoid smell temptations such as the bakery counter and the deli.

10 Eat
Best tip of the lot because, when it comes to weight loss, eating too little is your biggest enemy. Apart from testing your willpower to the extreme, eating too little puts your body on red alert, slows down your metabolism and apart from making you horribly cranky, also stops weight loss. Aim to eat something small every four hours.

11 Try grazing
If you're forever battling against your hunger pangs, think about grazing on small snacks. This not only keeps your blood sugar stable, so you'll suffer from fewer energy dips, but also stops you from reaching for something sugary for energy. Though be careful what you eat, not all snacks are made the same. Think a portion of dried fruit, cottage cheese, oatcakes, chocolate rice cakes or unsalted nuts.

12 Don't distract yourself while you eat
Eating your meals while chatting on the phone, watching TV or reading a magazine is a sure way not to notice you've eaten, and leave yourself feeling cheated and hungry for more. Limit your distractions, and you'll not only eat slower (allowing your stomach to register the fact it's no longer hungry) but also enjoy the process.

13 Pig out selectively
If you choose foods that have fewer calories, such as lean meats, vegetables and fruits, you can afford to eat a larger meal than someone who is eating a pizza. Also if you're going to break your diet, break it on something you enjoy, and slowly savour the taste without feeling guilty afterwards.

14 Take Sunday off
You don't have to diet seven days a week to lose weight. Watch what you eat six days a week and you can afford to treat yourself (that's treat, not eat your

body weight in food in one day) on a Sunday. This way you won't feel as if you are on an endless treadmill with no salvation in sight.

15 Think about what you're eating

Before you eat something, think about what the label means. 'Thirty-three per cent less fat' means 67 per cent fat (hardly low). 'Low fat' doesn't mean low calorie or low in sugar. 'Reduced' and 'lite' mean practically nothing and 'added vitamins' doesn't necessarily mean healthy.

16 Drink before you eat

Thirst signals are very close to hunger signals, which means often when we reach for food we should really be reaching for water. It's the old 1.5 litres a day trick. If you can't fathom that, carry a small bottle of mineral water around with you and keep topping it up until drinking becomes second nature.

17 Don't be afraid to throw away leftovers

Yes it's wasteful, but if it will stop you eating when you're bored it's worth it. One successful dieter suggests throwing away tempting foods into the bin, without their wrappers on to stop you retrieving it with rubber gloves at a later date.

18 Don't deny yourself delights

It's simple psychology: ban all chocolate and all you'll think about is chocolate, chocolate and chocolate. Better to give yourself one small bar a day so you won't dream about it at night.

19 Everything counts

Don't fall into the – 'What's the point in saying no to another cookie, I'm fat anyway?' trap. When it comes to diet and exercise, everything counts. Bad news on the diet front but good news on the exercise front, so balance it out.

20 Fat is good

You can't afford to cut all fat from your diet. Unsaturated fat can aid weight loss by turning off hunger signals. The fats to take are omega 3 and 6 essential fatty acids found in oily fish, nuts and seeds. Avoid saturated fat found in meat, butter and hard margarine.

chapter 3

Sculpt, stretch and de-stress

Question: what did your mum always tell you to do and you never did?

Answer: stand up straight!

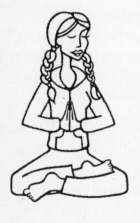

If you can stand up straight, you can work a room, make people notice you, even wear a potato sack and still look fabulous. You can even weigh what you want and look pounds lighter. Fabulousness aside, getting your posture right can also relieve numerous health issues, such as a bad back, PMS, flagging energy and sore limbs, which makes it a must if your aim is to look good. I know what you're thinking, a whole chapter devoted to posture – how hard can it be? Well, if you can do it properly it's not hard at all, but if you suffer from any of the above the chances are you need a helping hand.

Sculpting your body into good posture is all about making your muscles lean and long (as opposed to short and compact, which happens when you sit down all the time, wear high heels and generally lie slumped in front of the TV). Do it right and you will appear taller, slimmer, and more defined. You'll also look regal when you walk into a room and give off the air of someone filled to the brim with confidence. If this is your aim, then this is your chapter. Though bear in mind, sculpting alone won't help you lose weight, as it's not aerobic and, therefore, won't burn fat. And while certain types of yoga and Pilates will help you build lean muscle mass and shape up, it's the advanced variety that has to be done about three times a week, not the exercises below. This means if your aim is to lose weight and build a strong muscular body, this chapter works best if you combine it with 30 minutes of cardiovascular work from Chapter 4 or exercises from Chapter 5, or if you're feeling very committed, the bikini-fit plan in Chapter 6.

tip

Like it or not, good posture is the key to looking fabulous.

Who needs sculpting help?

You need sculpting help if you do or suffer any of the following (and it's not caused by a specific injury):

Lower back pain

It feels like someone's kicked you in the back and makes you want to slouch. This is usually the direct result of having little or no stomach muscles. This means the muscles in your lower back not only have to support the back but also the front of you as well.

Solution: you need to build up your core strength (see below).

Neck pain

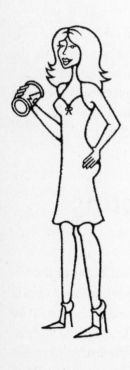

It feels like you can't turn your neck from left to right and it can give you headaches and sore shoulders. These days most of us have neck pain, the result of too many hours spent in front of a computer. Stand badly and it's likely you sit badly too. Osteopaths note that most of us end up letting computers suck our heads towards the screen in a kind of ostrich-neck look, where our chin juts forwards pulling our necks out of alignment and causing sore necks.

Solution: better seated posture.

You wear high heels

It feels like there are pins in the balls of your feet, and your calves are too tight. Posturally this makes you lean forwards and stick your bum out. The body in its natural state is beautifully designed to stand upright. However, the foot is the body's shock absorber; throw it off balance with high heels (that's 7.5cm (3in) or more) and it's virtually impossible to maintain good posture. This is because heels throw your body weight forwards leading to lower-back pain and possible injury to the discs.

Solution: wear high heels only for special occasions, and when you do, hold yourself upright from your centre (i.e., use your stomach muscles).

You balance more on one leg than the other when standing

It feels like you have one hip stuck out, and it can make one side of your body stronger and less flexible than the other. If you stand like this you're not alone. Most people have one side of their body that is stronger than the other (usually the side you write with). This causes an imbalance in the body where you can no longer tell whether you're standing straight, making you twist your pelvis and back.

Solution: stand in front of a full-length mirror and then stand sideways on and look at your alignment. Knees should be soft, stomach in, and legs straight, shoulders back, and head upright, all with no pain.

You can't touch your toes

You feel your back hurting the moment you try to reach towards the floor with your knees straight. You should be able to touch your toes easily without forcing your body or straining. The stretch doesn't come from your arms but from how flexible your lower back is. If your usual position is horizontal, and your idea of exercise is walking to the fridge, your muscles may be too tight to do this stretch.

Solution: take up some exercise. Flexibility is as important as strength and stamina.

You have a floppy belly even when you're standing tall

You feel you can't pull your stomach in. You haven't used your stomach muscles for so long some have switched off. The abdominals are a wider set of muscles than you think. There are three layers and the sit-up only works the upper two layers, plus if you have a layer of flab over these, no matter how hard you work they won't show through at all.

Solution: build up your core strength and do some fat-burning exercise.

You slump forwards the minute you sit down

You are generally more comfortable letting your body slump. You are so used to having bad posture that your body can't remember how to hold itself up properly, meaning when you try it's a strain and feels uncomfortable.

Solution: you need to retrain your body how to hold itself up.

You have shoulders that reach your ears

This is a stress response, and equals tight shoulders and a tight neck. Consciously pull your shoulder blades down your back (imagine them sliding down towards your waist); if you suddenly feel space around your neck, you've been walking around with your shoulders tensed up.

Solution: you need to work your upper back and train your lats (the bits under your arms) to pull down naturally.

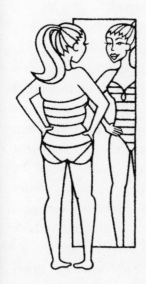

Get to grips with your core

Do you have a persistent ache in your shoulders, a tight, pulling feeling in your neck, a lower back that twinges and complains if you stand too long? If so, you're not alone. More than two in five people have experienced back pain lasting for more than one day. For half of these people, the pain lasted for more than four weeks.

While there are a variety of reasons why back problems occur, the most common is the lazy girl special: a combination of bad posture and inactivity. Or rather, long days spent slumped over a computer and nights spent slumped in front of the TV. This kind of sedentary lifestyle means your back and stomach muscles become severely under-used and generally get floppy. In many cases the stomach

tip

If you've been lucky enough to escape the agony of a bad back so far – don't fool yourself that you're immune. Statistics show back pain can affect anyone, men as much as women, young people as well as the old, the fit, the unfit, and even royalty.

muscles cannot then support the stomach and so the spine takes over and you get back pain. Roughly translated this means if you don't start moving and looking after your back one day soon, you're going to bend over and, wham! – a disc will rupture and your back will go into spasm.

The good news is there are preventative measures, and they're all to do with easy-peasy lifestyle changes.

Step 1: *work on your stomach*

You'll be wasting your time doing any of the above if, as many osteopaths and physiotherapists are now saying, you neglect to strengthen your core muscle groups: the transverses abdominis (known as your TVAs or abdominal muscles) and the diagonal obliques. These are the muscles that support your back and run around the body like a corset. New research from Queensland University shows that building strength here is essential for a much-coveted flat stomach. Research also shows that the core muscle groups need to engage automatically, but just one bout of back pain can switch them off, and the only way to switch them back on again is to exercise the muscles in the right way.

The way to do this is to pull in the lowest layer of stomach muscle without using the top two:

1. Lie on your back. Breathe in, place your hand on your belly button and, on the out breath, pull your stomach and lower abdominals in.

2. Imagine your belly button being pulled back towards your spine or the floor. If you feel your ribs contracting or the skin crease above your belly button you're sucking in too hard.

3. The aim is to build good endurance in this muscle so that it starts to pull in without you thinking when you walk, run or sit up. Do it three times a day for a flat tummy.

myth

Crunches and sit-ups are the best way to strengthen your middle. Untrue (see below) – the best way to get a strong core is to learn how to utilise all three layers of your abdominals, not just the surface six-pack layer.

Step 2: do some exercise

The facts are clear that most people suffer back pain between the ages of 20 and 40 because this is the time they put on weight and spend more time sitting than exercising. To combat this you need to do some exercise three to four times a week for at least 40 minutes (see below for specific exercises).

Your exercise regime should break down into 20 minutes of aerobic exercise – fast walking, running or cycling – ten minutes of good stretching and ten minutes of strengthening with weights (see Chapter 3 and 5). For rehabilitation, mobilisation and good posture, try Pilates, yoga and swimming (though don't swim with your head out of the water, as it strains your neck). Remember: if you suffer from very bad back pain be aware that you should see your doctor before starting any exercise regime. Plus, always tell gym staff and instructors about your back, and stop if you get a sharp pain.

Step 3: lose weight

Statistics show women on average gain almost 4.5kg (10lb) between the ages of 30 and 45 years, and two more between 45 and 55 years. While the weight itself won't damage your back, it will weaken your stomach muscles and reduce your overall chances of looking and feeling great. The way to tell if this is happening to you is to either stand up or climb some stairs. If you had to brace yourself to do either and/or can't see your toes when you look down, you need to lose some weight.

Step 4: be aware of your posture

The truth is most of us have no idea how to stand with good posture. If someone says stand up straight it's likely you suck in your stomach, puff out your chest and let your chin poke out. If this sounds familiar, it's worth noting that the spine is not naturally straight, and if you're standing correctly, there should be a gentle natural curve in the small of your back. To achieve this, think about standing tall, feet hip-width apart (your hips are smaller than you

tip

It's also important to think about how you do everyday things, such as sitting, standing and bending. Never throw yourself into a chair when you sit down, or brace yourself when you get up (use your stomach muscles and other muscle groups).

think) and imagine there is a string pulling you up from the centre of your head. At the same time keep your head in line with your spine and tuck your chin in, as if you were going for a double chin. Your stomach should be firm but not sucked in so you can't breathe, and your back should feel loose, not rigid.

myth

The best cure for a bad back is rest. Untrue, research shows backs get better a lot quicker if you keep them mobile.

Back-pain myths

Myth: *back pain is cured only by surgery.*

Truth: the majority of back pain is cured with physical treatment and lifestyle changes (only 5 per cent of cases are dealt with by surgery).

Myth: *pregnancy and back pain go hand in hand.*

Truth: as long as you keep your back moving with exercise, such as Pilates, your back won't cause you pain during pregnancy.

Myth: *sex and bad backs are a no-go.*

Truth: as long as you avoid bearing the weight of your partner, sex is fine. Go for an on-top position or side by side.

Myth: *sitting is bad for back pain.*

Truth: not if you sit correctly – with your legs, hip-width apart, and with support coming from your stomach.

20 minutes to a sculpted body

The following lazy girl exercise plans have been devised by experts and can be done anywhere, from the gym to your bedroom floor, and even in front of your TV.

Pilates

Does your fabulously un-flat belly block out the view of your feet and stop you from shoehorning yourself into your new jeans? If so, help is at hand with our fantastic belly-busting exercise plan based on Pilates (and devised by a Pilates teacher). Try it and it will turn even the wobbliest tummy into a washboard.

Pilates (pi-lah-tes) is a body-conditioning technique that is famously used by actors and dancers to create a long, lean, sculpted body. A gymnast called Joseph Pilates devised Pilates over 80 years ago, and it is based on

tip

Pick one set of exercises from the following section. Or pick and mix a few of the exercises. Repeat your chosen section three times a week. If you have an injury, always see your doctor first and stop if you feel a sharp pain.

working the deep 'core' postural muscles /
regularly and not only will you improve
also you'll be stronger, leaner and more toned.

Exercise one:

1. Lie on the floor on your back and put your fingertips just above your pubic bone (this is below your belly button). Now slowly lift your head off the floor and you'll feel your abdominal muscles pop up towards your fingers.

2. Put your head back down and repeat, *but* this time as you lift your head, draw your tummy muscles and navel back and upwards towards your spine to stop them from popping out (this is called your stomach connection, and if you want to work towards a flat stomach this should be used throughout all the exercises in this chapter, and Chapters 4, 5, and 6).

3. Repeat five to ten times. Each time try to find a deeper and deeper connection.

4. To enhance the effect, pout your lips (as if you were going to apply lipstick) and exhale in this position as you lift your head, as this will engage other muscles in your stomach area.

Fabulously works: your pelvic-floor strength, and helps give you a flatter stomach.

Exercise two:

This exercise can be done any time, from an advert break between TV programmes or when you're waiting for your bath to fill up.

1. Sit on the floor with your knees bent and feet flat. Grab a cushion, fold it in two and put it between your thighs. Make sure you have the stomach connection that you made in Exercise One before you start.

2. Squeeze the cushion with your thighs and push up on to the balls of your feet and then squeeze back down on to your heels. Repeat ten times.

3. Keep the cushion in the same place and repeat the exercise ten times, but this time with your toes touching and your heels apart.

4. With the cushion in the same place and feet flat on the floor, put your hands behind your head and roll your spine backwards until you are slouched in your favourite 'lazy girl' couch position, and then slowly roll that shape back up in a C-shaped curve. The trick is to squeeze the cushion hard between your thighs to pull yourself up. Repeat ten times.

5. Once you've become super fabulous at that, try curling up and down in a diagonal – i.e., your right shoulder to left knee and vice versa. Make sure your knees and hips stay pointing squarely in front of you.

Fabulously works: the inner thighs, and will whittle down your waist.

Exercise three:

1. Put the cushion behind your shoulders, lie back and stretch your arms back over your head so you open out your abdominal and

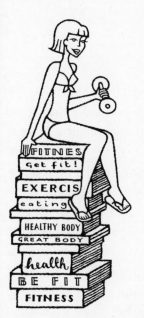

chest area. Your tailbone should be on the floor, your knees bent and your feet flat and belly button pulled in.

2. Assume the lazy girl position with your hands behind your head; now, keeping your shoulders relaxed (not up around your ears), pull up into a sit-up. Don't yank your head forwards, instead drop it into your hands and pull up from your stomach. At the top of your stretch, hold the position and try to pull your belly button further in as you breathe. Slowly drop back and repeat ten times.

Fabulously works: your stomach, and stretches your neck and back.

Exercise four:

1. Sitting on the edge of the sofa, put both hands either side of you and dip your hips off the sofa, with your knees bent and feet on the floor. Then drop your head towards your knees in a C-shape and feel your shoulders stretching (keep pulling that stomach in).

2. Then, pushing away from your arms, move back to a seated position, and repeat five times.

Fabulously works: your flabby underarms, and stretches your neck and shoulders.

Exercise five:

1. Lie on your back on the floor and place your arms out at the sides at shoulder level, point your toes and breathe in. Now as you exhale pull your belly button to your spine and hold it there.

2. Lift your right leg and, keeping it straight, make a giant circle (keeping your back on the floor). Make sure you lift up across the body and as near to the floor as possible and back to the starting position. Repeat five times on each leg.

Fabulously works: your tummy, legs and bottom.

Yoga

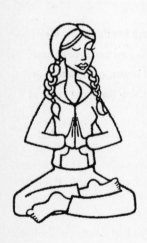

Whether you've dabbled with yoga before, or not, it's worth knowing that these days it's no longer the hippy, spiritual alternative to going to the gym but a serious workout designed to keep your body fit for life, no matter if you're young, old, flabby or fit. From a health perspective the benefits move well beyond a flexible body. One study carried out by the Department of Complimentary Medicine at the University of Exeter found yoga can help people manage and ease symptoms of chronic conditions, such as asthma and arthritis. Other pros, say the British Wheel of Yoga, include: improved flexibility and strength, an easing of muscle pain and improved digestion. Apart from helping with weight loss, yoga can also improve your stamina, help combat stress, tone and firm a flabby midriff, and improve your circulation and breathing capacity. Like Pilates, anyone can do it.

Exercise one:

1. Breathe in and stand with your feet close together and your arms by your side, balancing your weight evenly across your body. Breathe out and imagine a piece of string pulling you upwards from the top of your head, and one pulling you down from between your legs.
2. Breathe in again, let your stomach expand outwards, and breathe out, letting your stomach flatten. Each time you breathe, imagine the whole of your body relaxing and letting go.
3. Repeat ten times.

Fabulously works: on relaxing your entire body from head to toe.

Exercise two:

1. Sit down in front of the TV and breathe in, lifting upwards from your centre (again imagine your belly button travelling back towards your spine). Now breathe out and bring the soles of your feet together, and then let your legs flop outwards and your knees and thighs go soft, and either hold your feet or place your hands on your thighs.
2. Breathe deeply (as above) ten times.

Fabulously works: on loosening your hip flexors, your hips and strengthening your hamstrings (the bits down the back of your thighs).

> ## *tip*
>
> Never force a yoga move. Go as far as you can easily go – with time your body will stretch further and further.

Exercise three:

Famously known as the downward dog pose, this is really an inverted V-shape and is easier to get into if you start on all fours, keeping your arms shoulder-width apart, and your legs hip-width apart.

1. Stretch your arms out and place your palms face down on the floor. Now breathe in and, keeping your arms straight, lift up on to your feet (pulling in your stomach), and straighten your legs.
2. Breathe out and, keeping your head aligned with your back, imagine your bottom pointing up towards the ceiling and your head pointing towards the ground.
3. Breathe for ten counts and relax.

Fabulously works: the upper body, the arms and your stomach.

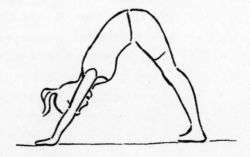

Exercise four:

1. Lie face down on the floor with your arms by your side, palms facing upwards and your legs together.

2. Now, keeping your stomach pulled in to support your back, lift your head and chest off the floor (imagine your head and chest pulling away from your body in a diagonal line).

3. Hold for three counts and repeat five to ten times. To help yourself, squeeze your thighs together as you lift.

Fabulously works: on opening up the chest area, strengthening the upper back and abdominals.

Types of yoga classes to try:

Astanga yoga: often described as power yoga, Astanga is the most physically demanding form of yoga. It's also the most cardiovascular because it's based around a dynamic continuous flow of movements and postures. Classes are fast and challenging so it's best to familiarise yourself with other forms of yoga before you try this.

Hatha yoga: this is the generic term for yoga and all other types of yoga are developed from this. It's the most widely available form and excellent for beginners. It is perfect if your body and mind are feeling over-stressed.

Sivananda yoga: this is still Hatha yoga but with a greater spiritual emphasis. It's based on a specific order of 12 positions and has a strong meditative element, which is good for people suffering from anxiety and depression.

Iyengar yoga: Iyengar is the most structured form of yoga. It focuses on getting every detail of every posture absolutely correct to enhance posture and body alignment. There is a strong remedial element, so it's excellent for stress, back pain, and high blood pressure.

Kundalini yoga: Kundalini is about breathwork and relaxation reached through a series of postures. It's also a way, say experts, to turn back the clock and erase the years. The guru behind this form of yoga, Gurmykh Kaur Khalsa, is 57 years old (and looks as if she is in her late thirties). 'Do Kundalini,' she says, 'and you never have to grow old'.

Bikram yoga: the central principle of Bikram yoga is that heat will help aid movement, flexibility and breathing. For this reason classes take place in rooms heated to around 38°C (100°F). The aim is also to help the body sweat out toxins and allow muscles to stretch fully.

The gym stuff — at-home sculpting work

If you've been doing the traditional sit-up and getting nowhere fast, it's simply because it engages the wrong tummy muscles. Luckily, American exercise scientist, Dr Peter Francis from San Diego State University, tested the 13 most popular abdominal gym exercises for effectiveness and came up with the top four belly busters.

Do three sets of all four exercises every day for 15 minutes to fabulously work your stomach.

The bicycle

1. Lie on the floor with your lower back pressed into the ground.
2. Put your hands behind your head. Bring your knees up to a 45-degree angle and slowly move your legs in a bicycle motion, while alternately touching your left elbow to your right knee, and your right elbow to your left knee.

Knee raises

1. Sit on the edge of a stable chair, knees bent, and feet flat on the floor; hold on to the sides of the chair.
2. Tighten your tummy, lean back slightly and lift your feet several inches off the floor.
3. Now in a steady movement pull knees in towards your chest and crunch your upper body forward. Lower your feet to the original position, and repeat.

Army sit-up

1. Lie down, knees bent, feet together and anchored under a steady couch. Loop a towel around the back of your neck and hold each end.
2. Contract your tummy (keep your belly button pulled to your spine) and curl upwards, lifting your shoulders, head and back,

curling all the way up, and then lower almost to the floor and repeat. If it's too hard, just lift your upper body off the floor and build up to the above.

Ball lift

1. Lie back, holding a tennis ball in your hands, and raise your arms towards the ceiling, with your legs extended together and feet flexed.
2. Tighten your tummy muscles and bottom and lift your shoulders and head a few centimetres (inches) off the ground. Make sure the ball goes towards the ceiling and not forwards.
3. Lower 2.5cm (1in), and repeat.

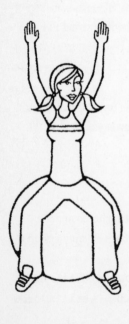

Swiss-ball work

1. A Swiss ball (also known as the stability ball/fitball and physioball) is that large brightly coloured, inflated ball that you probably see rolling about your local gym floor. The idea is that as the ball is full of air it has an unstable surface, so when you're sitting or lying on it and working major muscle groups, the smaller less-used muscles are also forced to work hard, to balance and stabilise the major muscles. Meaning you get a more intense and powerful workout.
2. It's harder than it looks, as the ball wobbles every time you move. Stop using your stomach muscles and you'll fall off, but fabulous for a toned, sexy flat stomach.

Handy hints:

Swiss balls come in small, medium and large. Opt for a medium sized ball unless you're super tall, and make sure you buy a good-quality ball that has been tested to high standards so it won't burst when you bounce up and down on it. Also be sure to pump it up to the right volume – the ball shouldn't sink when you sit on it.

Exercise one:

1. Lie on your left side on the ball, with your hip resting on top of the ball and your legs in a straight line resting on the floor. To make it easier, put your left leg in front of your right or place it against a wall for support.
2. Now, pulling in your stomach muscles, place your hands behind your head and slowly bend over the ball towards the floor, and then lift up to start position.
3. Repeat ten times and swap sides.

Fabulously works: your waist.

Exercise two:

1. Sit up on the ball with your feet flat on the floor. Let the ball roll slowly back, and slowly walk your feet forwards, and let your body slide down the ball until your thighs are parallel with the floor.

2. Your upper body should be resting on the ball. Hold yourself steady by pulling your stomach in (navel to spine).

3. Now cross your arms in front of your chest and lift your upper body forwards into a C-shape and return to start position.

4. Repeat ten times.

Fabulously works: your whole stomach and back.

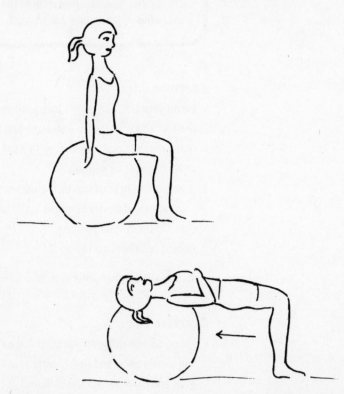

Exercise three:

1. Sit on top of the Swiss ball and place your legs hip-width apart. Now, pulling your stomach in (see Pilates section on how to do this properly), lift one leg off the floor (keeping both hips on the ball) and hold for five counts.
2. Repeat on the other leg, and then repeat ten times. If you feel you're going to fall, hold your arms out for balance (keeping your shoulders pulled down).

Fabulously works: your core.

tip

Don't be too adventurous on a swiss ball – it's easy to fall off when you're a beginner.

Exercise four:

1. Kneel with the ball in front of you. Lie your body over it, so your arms are on the floor in front of you.
2. Now slowly walk yourself forwards on your arms so that the ball rolls underneath you and you're supported by your straight arms. Your knees and legs should be resting on the ball.
3. In this position imagine you're as straight as a plank of wood and, holding your stomach in, bend your arms into a press-up.
4. Repeat and work to ten.

Fabulously works: your core and flabby underarms.

20 fabulous body tips

1 Breathe
Not only when you're doing stretching exercises (the power comes from the breath, so don't think so hard you forget to breathe), but also in everyday life. Studies show most of us forget to breathe or don't breathe fully (meaning we don't then relax fully) when we're stressed.

2 Breathe properly
The correct way to breathe for relaxation and during exercises is in through your nose, letting your stomach rise up when you breathe in, and imagining the breath filling your lungs with air. To breathe out make a 'shhh' noise through your mouth and soften from the stomach and all along the chest bone.

3 Don't shoulder the work
It's easy to let your shoulders do all the work your abdominals should be doing. Try the above exercises, and if you can't feel anything, start again by dropping your shoulders (so that the shoulder blades feel as if they are sliding down your back), then engaging your stomach muscles and then doing an exercise.

4 Don't cheat on stretching
Want long, slender, sexy limbs? Then always stretch both before and after exercising (or lying on the couch). Breathe deeply into a stretch and always hold for 45 seconds or it's a waste of your time.

5 Don't work it every day
Like all muscles, your stomach muscles need time to rest and get stronger. When you strength-train you break down muscle fibres, which the body then rebuilds, so it's stronger the next time it's challenged. This process takes 48 hours, which is why you need rest time.

6 Don't overdo it
There's a reason you need to do only three sets of ten (or less). If you're doing it right then you shouldn't be able to do more than 10–30 reps (though obviously

as you get stronger you can do more). Overdo it and you're more likely to cause some damage to the body.

7 Find the right back position

When you're lying on the floor your spine shouldn't be flat and pushed into the floor. You need to find what Pilates teachers call the neutral position: pull your belly button backwards and maintain a natural curve in the spine (you should be able to get your hand under your back while lying down).

8 Banish your love handles

Even if you do these exercises religiously for three months, if you still chow down on Mars bars for dinner, don't watch your diet and/or rarely do some aerobic exercise, your toned muscles will never see the light of day.

9 Stand on one leg

This is the perfect test for balance and posture. If you have good posture, you should be able to balance perfectly on each leg without wobbling.

10 Stretch at your desk

If you spend all day in front of a computer, you need to stretch every 45 minutes (at least), as sitting compresses the spine. If you can't get up and walk around, lace your hands together behind your back and let your shoulders drop. Then stand up, lace your fingers together in front of you (palms facing outwards), lift your arms above your head and drop your head forwards.

11 Think about the Alexander Technique

If your posture needs serious help, think about the above technique, which helps teach you correct posture when standing, sitting, lying down and even brushing your teeth. It's excellent for back problems, and devotees swear it makes them feel lighter and taller.

12 Measure your height

If you're shorter than you used to be, it indicates posture problems. See an osteopath and start doing the above exercises.

13 Think about your bra straps

If your shoulder straps keep falling down (and you're wearing the right bra size) it's an indication that your shoulders are rounded from hunching. If only one strap falls down, it's a sign you're weight isn't evenly distributed and you're probably bearing down harder on one side (very common).

14 Find an osteopath

Think of an osteopath like a car mechanic and book yourself in for regular MOTs on your back and joints. An osteopath can help with back pain, sports injuries and even headaches, as well as advise on posture and alignment issues.

15 Reach for the wall

If you stand an arm's length away and then stretch towards the wall, your hands should hit it at the same time. If not, your body is not aligned. Check your feet are hip-width apart and level, pull your stomach in, drop your shoulders and chest, and try again.

16 De-bloat your tummy

Don't be a wheat freak – too much refined carbohydrate (anything with white flour, such as bread and pasta) will soak up fluid and then jam up your insides giving you a tummy as tight as a drum. Reduce your intake or cut out for one week to see the difference.

17 Exercise in front of a mirror

Essential for posture and sculpting exercises to ensure you have the right posture and alignment. Look to make sure your feet are in parallel, your shoulders are dropped and your face is relaxed (this instantly relaxes your neck and shoulders).

18 Get to know your body

The next time you're slobbing on the sofa, feel around your body and find your tight spots. Dig in with your fingers to find the areas that won't give (a healthy muscle should give) and sore points that need to be relaxed. Then every day for ten minutes, lie on the floor and, breathing deeply, visualise these areas loosening and relaxing.

19 Have a massage

Forget body rubs, which lull you into a gentle sleep, these days massage has a more powerful health message to pummel home. Recent medical research shows that apart from diminishing aches and pains, massage can boost circulation, decrease levels of stress hormones, balance the nervous system and stimulate the nerves that supply blood to the muscles and major organs, helping you to feel glowing with health and energy.

20 ... and relax

For ten minutes each day, lie down. First breathe deeply then bend your knees to your chest and hold for two minutes as this helps stretch your spine. Let go and stretch your legs out – relax for eight minutes. We guarantee you'll feel taller and more refreshed when you get up.

chapter 4
Move your butt

OK, this is the chapter you never thought you'd be reading, the one where you have to accept that if you want to look fabulous you have to lift something heavier than the remote control and do more than take that daily stroll from your desk to the coffee machine. If you haven't done anything since you were forced to do cross-country runs at school, the chances are exercise is not currently a word in your vocabulary (or perhaps in your mind).

Maybe you're still convinced you're the glamorous party-girl type, not the health freak who would rather do aerobics than go shopping. Or maybe you feel at your age it's ungraceful to sweat or humiliating to admit to friends and family that you need to exercise. The good news is these days everyone – no matter what their shape, and/or age – should be exercising for the sake of their health and well-being. That's not just taking the stairs when you can be bothered but actually getting breathless three to four times a week for 30 minutes.

Whatever your excuse (oops, sorry, reason), if your aim in reading this guide is to increase your overall fitness levels, then this is the chapter for you. (For a total body re-haul see Chapter 6, to tone up your troublesome zones see Chapter 5, and to stretch and shape see Chapter 3).

Exercise three times a week and you will:

- Feel toned and honed.
- Have more energy.
- Have better skin.
- Have more stamina.
- Lose weight.
- Have muscle definition.
- Be in a better mood.
- Be better in bed.
- Improve your overall health.
- Have fewer colds.
- Sleep better.
- Eat better.
- Have more confidence.
- Have better self-esteem.
- And look fantastic.

What shape are you in?

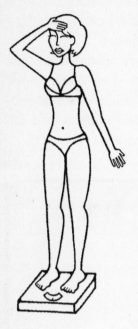

Before you start, it pays to know your personal starting line. You might be honest enough to admit that your stomach could do with some work, and that you practically have a heart attack when you have to run for a bus, but what shape are you really in? Try the following tests to work out what areas you need to be focusing on:

Flexibility

How bendy you are is essential, as healthy muscles need to stretch and lengthen as you move, otherwise you'll be prone to injury, aches and pains.

Test: stand up straight, with your stomach pulled in (the right way to do this is to imagine sucking your navel backwards towards your spine and holding it there), chest dropped, and knees straight, and legs hip-width apart. Now slowly breathe in and, on the exhale, drop your head and bend, reaching your arms towards the ground, and see if you can touch your toes (no cheating, keep your knees straight and don't force the movement).

If you can't reach further than your knees – you need to focus on stretching and lengthening your muscles (see Chapter 3).

If you can reach your ankles – that's fabulous – you're bendy enough!

If you can easily put your hands on the floor – you're super flexible but probably need to work on your strength to help stabilise your body (Chapter 5).

Strength

Strength is vital not only for fitness but also for health, as all of us lose lean muscle mass and bone density as we get older, leaving us prone to osteoporosis (brittle-bone disease) and weight gain.

Test: try to do a press-up. Place your hands and feet on the floor and walk your legs back behind you. Now balance on your toes and place your arms shoulder-width apart, palms facing forwards and in line with your shoulders. Pull your stomach in so your body is in a straight line, and lower your body to the floor, and then push back up with your arms. Repeat for as long as you can.

If you can do only one – you need to focus on upper body training (see Chapters 3 and 5).

If you can do three to four – you need to focus on overall strength training (Chapter 5).

If you can easily do ten – go to the running section of this chapter to make sure your cardiovascular work is in line with your strength.

Stomach power

All types of exercise should enlist your core muscle groups – these are the muscles that surround your body like a corset. If you can't activate them you'll be prone to backache (as your back will be supporting your stomach) and fatigue every time you exercise or stand for long periods.

Test: do the plank. Get back into the press-up position, but this time keep your elbows on the floor and clasp your hands together. Now, pulling your belly button to your spine, lift your body off the ground (make sure you are holding your body in a straight line) and hold this position.

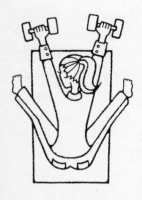

If you can hold this for less than six seconds or your back hurts – you need to focus on your abdominals (Chapters 3 and 5).

If you can hold this for 10–20 seconds before your back hurts, you need to practise pulling your abdominals in tighter, and strengthening your back (see Chapters 3 and 5).

If you can hold it for 25–30 seconds and your back doesn't hurt – you have fabulous abdominals.

Cardiovascular fitness (stamina)

Cardio is exercise that needs a high level of exertion and so requires a lot of oxygen, breathing and heart-pumping work. This is essential to lower your risk of a serious disease, burn body fat and generally keep you looking trim.

Test: put some running shoes on and, at a steady pace (too fast and you'll exhaust yourself), either run round your local park or your garden. (NB Be sure to warm your muscles up first by either jogging on the spot for a minute or stretching.)

If you can run for no more than five minutes – you need to boost your stamina; keep reading this chapter.

If you can run for ten minutes – you're doing well but could do with a boost; try the Bikini-fit plan in Chapter 6.

If you can run for 20 minutes – you're doing well and could do with challenging yourself with faster runs, or runs on an incline.

A lazy guide to getting fit

tip

How many days/ weeks/months/years have you been telling yourself you're going to get fit/lose weight/look fabulous? At a conservative estimate it's probably about a year, which means even if you'd only exercised for half of that time you'd be in shape by now.

If you want to lose weight and firm up, any change in your activity levels will help you burn off calories. This logically means, the more you do and the more sustained your effort (i.e., the more oomph you put in) the quicker the results. Here's how to start.

The non-exercise stuff

This is the stuff that is more essential than you think. Not just because it will help you get in shape but because exercise is more fun when you have a couple of props to throw around. What's more, buying workout gear doesn't have to cost you a fortune, but if you're stuck for cash or prefer to spend your money on other things, you can adapt what you already have hanging around your home and make use of them.

1 Home gym equipment

Stuff for the home gym is no longer expensive and it's available either through the Internet (so you don't have to lug it home) or in your local shop (see Resources for stockists). What's more it's not cumbersome, so when you're not using it you can hide it under your bed. To get quick results it pays to have a few (if not all) of the following:

A Swiss ball: (also known as the stability ball/fitball and physioball) is a large, brightly coloured, inflated ball that looks like a giant beach ball. The term was coined back in 1965 when a group of Swiss physical therapists started using it to work with injured and disabled people. As the ball is full of air, it has an unstable surface, so when you're sitting or lying on it and working the major muscle groups, the smaller less-used muscles are also forced to work, to balance and stabilise the major muscles. Meaning you get a more intense and powerful workout. The balls come in small, medium and large sizes, but you should opt for a medium size unless you're super tall. Also make sure you buy a good-quality ball that has been tested to high standards so it won't pop when you bounce up and down on it. Be sure to pump it up to the right volume – the ball shouldn't sink when you sit on it.

Weights/dumbbells: weights are available very cheaply everywhere and come either as hand-held weights, or strap-on weights that can be fastened around your wrists and ankles. You can even get inflatable weights; known as Aqua bells that are a bit like arm bands that need to be filled with water. Don't buy weights that are either too heavy or too light, as you'll end up not using them. The best sizes are 3–8kg. Go heavier if you want a tougher workout (see Chapters 5 and 6).

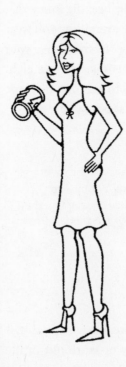

If you don't want to buy weights, think about using your food cupboard – tins, packets of sugar and flour, and empty plastic containers of milk (that you can fill with water) will also work, though won't be as accurate or heavy as proper weights.

A towel rolled up/small pillow: other versatile home products are towels and pillows or cushions (see Chapters 3 and 5 for exercises). These not only act as resistance for toning exercises but also can act as an unstable surface if you want to challenge yourself during toning, or as a head rest during the sculpting sessions.

2 Trainers

It's wise to focus the majority of your attention and money on footwear. This is just one reason why it pays to go to a specialist running shop, here they will not only take into account your gender (male and female feet are different, so

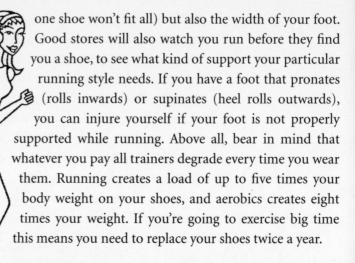

one shoe won't fit all) but also the width of your foot. Good stores will also watch you run before they find you a shoe, to see what kind of support your particular running style needs. If you have a foot that pronates (rolls inwards) or supinates (heel rolls outwards), you can injure yourself if your foot is not properly supported while running. Above all, bear in mind that whatever you pay all trainers degrade every time you wear them. Running creates a load of up to five times your body weight on your shoes, and aerobics creates eight times your weight. If you're going to exercise big time this means you need to replace your shoes twice a year.

myth

Always buy a well-known branded trainer. Wrong – don't be seduced by style trainers. If they look good on your feet they are often no use for running. Always buy your trainers from a specialist sports shop. See Resources.

3 Workout gear

What you wear can literally make or break your workout. If you know you're going to get sweaty or work out in the elements, look for clothes with labels saying: 'Dry Max/Dry Fit', 'Cool Max' and 'Supplex'. These all allow you to stay cool and dry no matter what kind of sport you're doing, as they draw moisture away from the body. Get used to reading the labels to see if the clothing you like supports the exercise of choice. For example, it's no use picking a loose pair of yoga leggings if your aim is to go running. Yoga wear is thicker than running wear, because it takes into account the slowness of the technique and the fact that the body cools down and needs to be kept warm.

myth

You don't need a proper sports bra. Wrong, a sports bra is an essential item. Tests show wearing a sports bra reduces breast movement by as much as 56 per cent, which will improve your workouts no end (and help you avoid breast pain).

Sportswear fabrics

Fabrics are divided into three areas when it comes to sportswear:

1. Fabrics that are worn next to the skin, and which transfer moisture away from the skin.
2. Insulating fabrics that retain heat.
3. Outer-shell fabrics that resist water and wind but still 'breathe', allowing moisture to pass through.

4 Find a personal trainer

A personal trainer is no longer the domain of the rich and famous, meaning they're more affordable than you think. Motivational aspects aside, a trainer can help you focus on the areas that annoy you the most, and push you to do the things you wouldn't do on your own. Sadly, there are a lot of untrained people out there saying they are personal trainers when they're not, which means you need to be careful whom you choose.

Before you start working with someone, always make sure they are trained. Look for a personal training diploma, degree, or relevant gym training (and make sure it's a gym you've heard of).

Next, ask questions: does he/she have insurance and first aid skills? What can you expect from sessions, and where has he/she worked before and for how long? Does he/she know what core strength is (a buzzword in fitness for using and building strong stomach muscles and using them in every type of exercise you do)?

Finally, go by your gut. You should have some kind of rapport with a trainer and not be afraid of him or her. If they make you feel intimidated, or don't ask you about your aims and goals, or give you the same thing to do without variation every single time you see them, feel free to look elsewhere.

tip

Having a trainer is a must if you're totally unmotivated, have no idea what you're doing and know from experience that you're likely to give up any exercise plan after a week.

5 Think about a gym

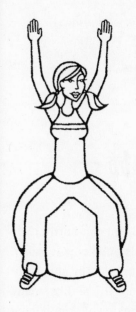

You don't have to join a gym to get in shape (see Chapter 6 for more details of a home plan), but it can help, especially if the sofa's too tempting every night. Like personal trainers, the gym you choose should be a carefully thought-out plan.

Pick a gym that you're likely to go to. It sounds obvious, but there's no point picking one next to your house if five days a week you're at work or out socialising. Likewise, there's no point in choosing one that's difficult to get to, because when you're tired and flagging you just won't go.

Always visit a number of gyms before you choose. This will help you to get a good idea of facilities and the kind of people who go there. Are you looking for a mixed gym, one that has a ladies' gym or one without children? What are the classes like? Do you get free towels? And will they write you a programme when you join?

Next, always read the small print. Lots of gyms have tie-in policies, so that even if you don't go you're signed up for a year and have to pay. This means it's important to be 100 per cent sure you will go, otherwise all you'll lose in a year is money (this happens to three in five people who join gyms).

Don't just go for the flash option – while it's nice to have a sauna, juice bar and steam room, your real focus should be classes and the gym. Look for a clean gym, equipment that's in good working order, a wide variety of classes at all levels, and also look for gym staff who do more than watch MTV.

myth

Gyms are full of super fit, Lycra-clad women and men running madly and pumping iron. Don't be gym prejudiced – the reality is somewhat different. Most gyms are full of people like you and me, and attract all levels of fitness, sizes and shapes.

The exercise stuff — running

Running is a huge calorie burner as you can burn nearly 500 calories in just 45 minutes; it also makes you leaner, sculpts your leg muscles, firms your bottom and is an amazing stress reliever. If, however, you're like many women out there, you're probably thinking of skipping the running bit because you're positive you can't run and probably have a couple of hundred excuses including:

- You were rubbish at it at school.
- You have weak ankles and knees.
- You're too self-conscious to try.
- You are too afraid to run alone.

- You worry that people will laugh at you.
- You're not the running type.

The simple fact is everyone can run, no matter what your PE prowess was at school or how much exercise you have done in the last five years. All it takes is preparation, effort and patience with yourself. Here's how to get your running legs on:

Don't run before you can walk

Before you even try to run you should be able to walk briskly for 30 minutes.

The aim with this (and with all cardiovascular work) is to workout at your training heart rate, which is between 60 and 75 per cent of your age-predicted maximum heart rate (APMHR).

However, the real trick is to exercise at an intensity where you can talk but feel breathless. If you feel you can't breathe, and you can't speak or are going to pass out, slow down because you're working too hard. If you can sing along to MTV and have a chat on your mobile then you need to work harder.

Stretch first

All it takes is ten minutes a day to increase flexibility, so, tempting as it is to skip stretching before you walk and run – don't! Think of your muscles like a new pair of tights.

tip

Running is just for the super fit isn't it? Well, not if you watch any of the world's marathon races. There you'll see people of all ages and sizes running for pure pleasure – last year as many as 34 million Americans ran for pleasure.

APMHR — how to work out your age-predicted maximum heart rate

To work this out take your age and subtract it from 220 (the Age-Predicted Maximum Heart Rate). This means that if you are 30 years old, your APMHR is 190 and your training heart rate zone is 114–142.

When you get new tights out of the packet, they are tight and compacted, so in order to get them on easily you first need to stretch them out. Likewise, when you exercise a muscle, or if you haven't exercised one for a while, it becomes tighter and shorter and gives you a limited range of movement. If you want a long, lean-muscled look you need to flex. Do it right and this will make the muscle more pliable and reduce your chance of injury.

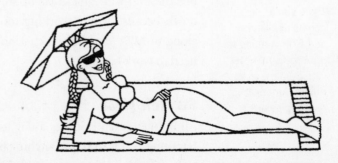

Do these stretches before running (and exercise workouts):

A calf stretch (your lower leg muscle):

1. Hold the wall for support (arm's length away), place hands at chest level and step back with the left foot; slightly bend the right leg.
2. Keep your back straight and your belly button pulled into your spine (this activates your stomach muscles) and push into the heel of your back leg.
3. Hold for 30 seconds and swap legs.

Hamstring stretch (the muscle than runs from your bottom to your thigh):

1. Lie on your back on the floor and bend your knees, keeping both feet on the ground. Lift one leg up straight and hold it behind the thigh with your hands, and then gently pull towards your chest.
2. Make sure you keep your tailbone (bottom) firmly on the ground so you can feel the stretch.
3. Hold for 30 seconds and swap legs.

Quad stretch (outer thigh muscle):

1. Stand in front of a wall and place one hand on the wall for support.
2. Now lift the opposite leg, and, holding the foot, bring that leg towards your bottom and hold for 30 seconds.

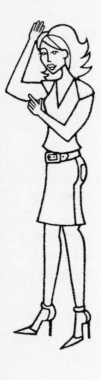

Hip stretch:

1. Lie on your back, with your arms stretched out to the side, now bend both legs at the knees with your feet on the floor.
2. Slowly roll the knees to the left until they are on the floor and hold for ten counts. This will stretch out your hip and waist. Then repeat on the other side for ten counts.

Triceps stretch (the flabby batwing bit under your arm):

1. Lift your left arm above your head (keep the shoulder down), now bend the arm, and let your hand fall behind your left shoulder.
2. Place your right hand on the elbow of the left arm and push down gently. You should feel a stretch in the back of the left arm.
3. Repeat five times and change arms.

Cat stretch:

1. Perfect for your back and chest. Kneel on your hands and knees.
2. Now round your back like a cat (make sure the curve comes from your chest bone and upper back) and then reverse it into an arch with your head and neck up.
3. Repeat five times.

Get your running technique right

- To walk effectively the most important fact to remember is always to walk heel to toe (obvious but not many people do it). This means as you take a step your heel should hit the ground first and your body weight should move through the foot into the toe (this is the same for running).

- Don't tense your upper body as you walk or run. This makes it harder to breathe and will reduce your stamina. Hold yourself from your stomach (belly button to spine) also known as your core, not from your chest, and imagine your upper body being loose and relaxed.

- Focus instead on looking out in front of you. It can help to imagine there is a piece of string pulling up from the top of your head all the way through your spine.

- Don't pound the ground. While running is a high-impact sport, you don't have to hit the ground with force (this can injure your knees). Again think upwards and release the tension in your upper body as you land.

- Let your arms swing. Keep elbows bent at 90 degrees but don't keep them fixed as this can hinder your running. The aim of the arms is to power your run, so use them to get momentum by pumping them as you run.

- Finally, when you run don't aim to bounce, or lift the feet too far off the ground and/or land on your toes. To run properly you should always land on your heels and use short, easy strides, not big, bounding ones.

tip

Avoid looking down as you run. The average head weighs 4.5kg (10lb), so looking down pulls your body out of alignment, and it will hurt your neck and shoulders.

Interval train

Beginners should always start with interval training, which, apart from being easier, helps build up your stamina levels. All it means is walking and then running and then walking again to recover your breath so you can run again. If you've never run before, it can take a leap of faith to try this and you may feel silly at first (which is why it helps to run with a friend or with a trainer). The solution here is just to take a deep breath, think of the benefits to your body and go for it (it also helps to run in the park where there are other people running). Believe us, after 30 seconds you'll be too focused on what you're doing to be worried about how you look.

The six-week running programme

Week 1:

Walk for 25–30 minutes.

Monday, Wednesday and Friday: walk for 25–30 minutes.

Pace: you should walk at a pace where breathing is difficult for you but not impossible. If you can talk but not have a fully blown conversation with someone, you're at the right intensity.

Week 2:

Walk and run for 30 minutes.

Monday, Wednesday and Friday: walk for two minutes,

run for two minutes, and repeat three times (for 12 minutes). Then walk for four minutes and run for two minutes and repeat three times (for 18 minutes).

Week 3:

Walk and run for 30 minutes.

Monday, Wednesday and Friday: run for three minutes, walk for two minutes and repeat three times (for 15 minutes). Then run for four minutes and walk for one minute, and repeat three times (for 15 minutes).

Week 4:

Run and walk for 30 minutes.

Monday, Wednesday and Friday: run for eight minutes, walk for two minutes and repeat three times (for 30 minutes).

Week 5:

Run and walk for 33 minutes.

Monday, Wednesday and Friday: run for ten minutes, walk for one minute, and repeat three times (for 33 minutes).

Week 6:

Run and walk for 35 minutes.

Monday, Wednesday and Friday: walk for two minutes, run for 15 minutes, walk for three minutes, run for 15 minutes (for 35 minutes).

tip

Feeling you can't run is a common fear. Most runners admit the first step was always the hardest, so don't give up.

As you get fitter you can increase the length of running and take shorter rests, so you are working harder for longer. Don't increase you running time above 35 minutes (unless you're training for a marathon), instead think about increasing the challenge:

1. Run with friends – this can enhance your performance and boost your motivation. find a running club near you by checking your local gym.
2. Run up hills for more of a challenge to your stamina.
3. Pick up the pace – running faster has mental benefits as well as physical payoffs. Try running for eight minutes and then adding one- or two-minute surges, slowing down and then repeating it again.
4. Run outside as well as at the gym – outside workouts work your thighs and bottom more than the treadmill.
5. Take a week off after a six-week programme, and when your body feels tired out.

More aerobic stuff

Can't convince you to run? Then make sure you incorporate one of the following into your life three times a week, making sure to challenge yourself (remember if you're not sweating or tired afterwards you haven't worked hard enough).

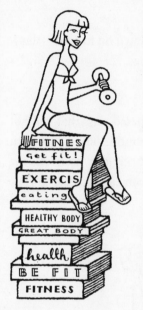

Walking

This improves cardiovascular (the way your lungs and heart work) strength and muscle strength. Plus it's cheap, it's easy and it can be done in high heels (good for calf strength, but we wouldn't recommend it).

Swimming

This improves upper- and lower-body muscles as well as aerobic strength and it's also cheap and can be easily done, though be sure to push yourself and not just float and glide for 30 minutes a day. One good way is to swim ten lengths, then use a paddle-board and swim another ten, focusing on your legs. Again swim for at least 20 minutes.

Cycling

This works the arms and legs and can actually be fun. If you want to work your bottom, keep your seat low, and don't rely on momentum to get you around, go at a steady pace, and challenge yourself with some hills.

Spinning class

Join a powerful 45-minute bike-based class with special stationary bikes that you pedal at different speeds and with different resistances, standing up and sitting down.

Step class/video

Involves literally stepping up and down on to a box (step); it's aerobic and fantastic for your legs.

Aqua aerobics

Powerful and very efficient water-based class that will not only tone the body but also burn around 500 calories in an hour. The benefits include fat burning, a boost to the metabolism, major resistance work and an increase in your heart and lung capacity.

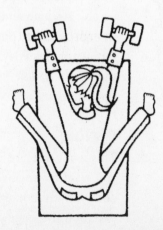

The best time to exercise

The time when you know you'll actually do it is usually the best time for exercise; for most people this means first thing in morning simply because they can get it over and done with. However, if you're not an early bird forget trying this, and if you rarely get a lunch hour, don't bother taking your gym kit to work. Instead, think of something you do every day without fail – for most people this is lounging around the house in the evenings, which makes this the ideal time to spend one hour exercising (see Chapters 5 and 6 for home tips).

In terms of your body's cycle the following times of day are best for certain results and personality traits:

7.00–9.00 a.m.: this is a good time to lose pounds, as most people exercise on an empty stomach, which forces your body to burn fat stores. An early morning workout will also kick-start your metabolism and keep you burning calories all day. One important fact: it's essential you warm up, as your joints will feel stiffer than at later times of the day.

12.00–2.00 p.m.: exercise before lunch, not afterward, otherwise you'll feel too sluggish to move. Make sure you've had breakfast and an 11.0 a.m. snack or else you'll literally be running on empty after working all morning, meaning you'll never make it to an hour.

3.00–5.00 p.m.: this is a good time to do competitive sports, as research shows this is when your co-ordination is at its highest, and your body is stocked up on energy from lunch and breakfast.

7.00–9.00 p.m.: peak time to exercise, as the body is warmed up and flexible, and as it's at peak temperature you'll have greater stamina, adrenaline and strength, meaning it's a good time to build muscle.

9.00–12.00 p.m.: your body's too tired – don't exercise!

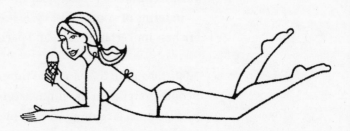

20 ways to keep moving

1 Remind yourself it can change the shape of your body

Nothing changes your shape as much as exercise – so while you can't make yourself taller or turn yourself into someone new, you can end up with a super-sexy, enviable body.

2 Keep an exercise journal

Not only will this spur you on but it will also help you to see how far you've come. Every time you work out, write down what you achieved and next time try to better your time, increase your repetitions or lift a heavier weight.

3 Take before and after pictures

There's nothing more motivating than seeing a photograph of yourself. If you don't want to weigh yourself, get a friend to take a photo of you every four weeks (preferably in the same outfit) and chart your change visually.

4 Get rid of that stitch

The first step is to eat an hour before exercising, and no later, so your stomach isn't heavy. Then while moving, sip; don't gulp water so that it overfills your stomach. To stop a stitch, pull your stomach muscles in tighter when you're running and breathe deeply into the side that hurts.

5 Exercise on your holidays

You don't have to go all out for runs, but if you want to avoid the inevitable holiday weight gain (this can be up to half a stone at Christmas time) make sure you keep active. Try going on hikes, swimming every day, and going for long, brisk walks.

6 Don't be a creature of habit

As tempting as it is to keep doing the same thing (because you're either good at it or you can't be bothered to change your routine) it pays to know that muscles adapt very quickly to what you're doing. This means every six weeks you need to do different things and keep challenging yourself.

7 Change your diet
Especially if your aim is to lose weight and tone up. While exercise does speed up the metabolism and help you lose inches, to lose fat and show off your new amazing muscles, you need to eat healthily.

8 Increase your protein count
Foods such as lean meats, cottage cheese and eggs will help boost the metabolism, especially if you're also working out. Reduce your saturated fats (cheese, fatty meats, cakes and biscuits) and you'll be laughing all the way to a size ten.

9 Play mental games
Promise yourself you'll stop when you've reached a certain distance or time, and then when you get there challenge yourself to do two minutes more, and keep going until you've had enough.

10 Wear a proper sports bra
Not just a support top. Studies from Edinburgh University show that even an A-cup moves 4cm (1½in) away from the ribcage during strenuous exercise leaving you at risk of ligament pain that will probably interfere with your running technique.

11 Use good technique
Don't hold on to the treadmill when running, yank your head up during sit-ups, lift weights too fast, or land on the balls of your feet as you run. All of these will hinder your results and could lead to an injury.

12 Think of weight loss
Intense exercise can sometimes suppress appetite, as there is a reduced blood flow to the digestive system, because activity draws blood to the muscles.

13 Think of your health
A new UK study shows that people who are unfit and overweight at 40 knock seven years off their life expectancy. By comparison researchers estimate for every hour of exercise you take, there is a two-hour increase in longevity to your life.

14 **Exercise to feel happy**
A study from University of New York medical school found those who regularly worked out were happier, less depressed and had fewer episodes of PMS than those who didn't.

15 **Remind yourself you're doing more than 58 per cent of people**
A study by the National Association for Sport and Physical Education found 88 per cent of women thought they were getting enough exercise but only 30 per cent were getting the recommended 30 minutes a day.

16 **Exercise to party harder**
It's the old use-it-or-lose-it theory. If you work out, you'll boost your mind and body's energy levels for up to 24 hours.

17 **Lower your blood pressure**
Good news for your heart, as high blood pressure is a major cause of strokes and heart attacks.

18 **Strengthen your bones**
All it takes is 20 minutes of weight-bearing exercise three times a week to strengthen your bones. This is anything that involves putting pressure on your bones; for example, jogging, walking and lifting weights.

19 **Lower your risk of breast cancer**
Breast cancer currently affects one in 12 women, but the good news is studies show that if you exercise four times a week, you can lower your risk by nearly 60 per cent.

20 **Exercise equals power**
Apart from keeping you healthy and happy – making exercise part of your everyday life will make you fitter, leaner and stronger than all your friends!

chapter 5

Shape up your flabby bits

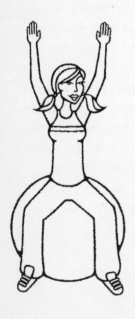

There are many ways to change your shape. You can throw yourself into a vigorous regime and radically change the whole of your body in a matter of months. You can take up a new sport, such as running, and watch how it changes your shape over time. Or you can target the area you hate the most and pummel it into shape (though note, unless you also change your diet too, you won't be able to trim an area down but simply firm it up). If shaping your flabby bits is your aim, then this is the chapter for you because we're talking batwing arms, wobbly bellies, thighs that jiggle long after you've sat down, and breasts that happily skim your lap. If this is your future (or more frighteningly your present) the facts are simple – do no exercise and your body will end up as firm as a plate of strawberry jelly. Here's just one good reason why you need to lift weights: to look good. However, before you envisage yourself pinned under an 18kg barbell or looking like the female equivalent of Mike Tyson, it's worth noting that the vast majority of women (and that's nearly 98 per cent of us) don't need to worry about developing man-sized biceps.

Better still, lifting weights is the perfect type of exercise for lazy girls, as you can do it in front of the TV or lying on your bedroom floor, which means it takes zero motivation compared to cardiovascular exercise, which, let's face it, means leaving the house. Strength-train properly, that is don't cheat on the repetitions, and we guarantee you'll lose body fat, speed up your metabolism and get a firmer and more fabulous physique. This happens because muscle is an active tissue (unlike fat which does nothing but make you look like a beached whale), so it basically eats up energy in your body. This means the more overall muscle you have, the more energy you will burn (meaning you can eat more food and not gain weight, or eat more healthily and lose weight).

myth

Weightlifting will turn me into the hulk. Untrue. Females have only one tenth of the muscle-building male hormone (testosterone) that men have, which means that no amount of lifting will bulk you out.

A strong muscular body also means:

- A lower risk of heart disease.
- Stronger bones (and less risk of osteoporosis when you're older).
- More energy – the stronger you are, the more your body can cope with on a daily basis.
- A better mood – thanks to an endorphin release from working out.
- A loss of inches – as muscle takes up less room than fat in the body.
- No age-related weight gain – after the age of 40 years 225g (½lb) of muscle is lost and replaced by fat.
- Better stamina.

Strength-training will help you:

- Lose weight – as muscles burn more calories than fat.
- Lose inches – as muscle takes up a third less space in the body than fat.
- Keep your body years younger. A study on older women from the College of Sports Medicine in the UK, found that those who lifted weights for a year had bodies that were 15 years more youthful than those who didn't.

Weight-training fears

Of course, it's hard to see this when the popular image of people using weights are guys who have no neck, can't put their arms down owing to over-developed arm muscles and generally grunt loudly every time they move. So for those who aren't yet convinced, let us dispel a few of your more common fears.

If I start exercising and then stop all my muscle will turn to fat. Untrue! Muscle and fat are different body tissues, which means if you stop exercising, you won't get fat because of muscle loss, but because you're burning less calories each day but still eating the same amount (this can add up to as much as 500 extra calories a day).

Why do some women look like body builders? These women are genetically placed to end up looking like this because they have a larger muscle mass than other women. Even then to get to this point they have to not only eat large quantities of protein to help build the muscle but also lift hefty (as in extremely heavy) weights for at least two hours every day. This is unlikely to be you, especially if your natural habitat is the sofa.

I worry that my thighs/arms/calves will become chunky if I weight train. Studies show we tend to exercise the parts of our bodies that are already strong because it's easier than challenging our weaker spots. If you therefore, keep doing something like the step or leg press because you're good at it, all you'll be doing is working your leg muscles to the extreme and bulking up. Variety is the name of the game.

I can't lift heavy weights so what's the point in lifting weights? Muscles grow by overloading the muscle fibres, and to overload them you don't have to lift 22.5kg (50lb) weights, but do a series of repetitions with light weights, which cause the muscle to 'burn' (ache). The fibres then repair themselves and get stronger once you have stopped, and that's how your muscles get stronger.

myth

Aerobics is better for reshaping your body than lifting weights. Untrue. Weight training boosts the rate at which you burn calories/energy and adds muscle to your body, which in turn changes your shape.

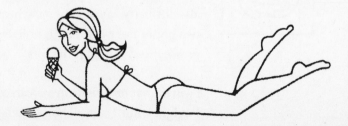

Targeting your trouble zones

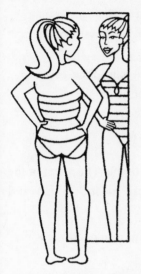

The beach season cometh (and sooner than you think)! Luckily, you can turn yourself from a cuddly couch potato to fabulous bikini babe by targeting your problem areas – starting right now. However, be realistic, if you need to target more than one zone, it's wiser to do the bikini-fit plan in Chapter 6, otherwise you will basically be exercising all the time.

Do all the exercises in your chosen category three times a week and remember these exercises work better if you combine them with 20–30 minutes of cardiovascular work (this will still equal only one hour's worth of exercise) three times a week and maintain a healthy diet.

Big flabby bottom

Want the derrière of a peach (rather than a watermelon)? Here's how:

Step-up:

1. This works your thighs, bottom, hips and calves. Place one foot in the middle of the first step of your stairs. Now, standing still, lift the other leg up so the knee is just above your hip and lower it back to floor. Repeat without resting (do this at a pace).

2. Do three sets of 15–20 repetitions. To make it more challenging hold 5kg (11lb) weights in each hand and increase your speed.

Stability bridge:

1. Lie on your back with your knees bent and both feet resting on an unstable surface, such as a rolled-up towel about 10cm (4in) high.
2. Now lift your hips off the floor (clench your bottom as you do this) and then slowly lower to the start position.
3. Repeat 15 times. Do three sets.

The lunge:

Top of its class for bum and thigh toning! The secret of the lunge lies in the fact it simultaneously tones the thighs and bottom.

1. Stand with your feet slightly apart, hold your tummy in (belly button to spine), place a weight in each hand and lunge (take a big step) forward.
2. As the front foot lands, bend the front knee so that your hips drop between your feet and your back knee goes down. Then push back to your starting position and repeat.
3. Do three sets of 15–20 repetitions, alternating between legs.

The static lunge:

Very similar to the above, the only difference being that once you have lunged forward you stay in position and move up and down (slowly) in a vertical movement.

1. Go down until the knee is a few inches off the floor then come up. Hold 5kg (11lb) weights in each hand to make it more challenging.
2. Do three sets of 15–20 repetitions on each leg.

The squat:

This is fabulous for a firm bottom.

1. Stand with your feet slightly wider than shoulder width. Imagine you're about to sit on a chair and, keeping your stomach pulled in and your back straight, literally squat down. Keep the knees in line with your toes at all times. Slowly return to start position and repeat. If you feel you're going to fall over, keep your arms stretched out in front of you for balance.
2. Do three sets of 15–20 repetitions.

Kneeling kick back:

1. Get down on all fours and pull your stomach muscles in. Raise your right leg off the floor and, with your knee bent, bring it into your body, then stretch it out backwards so that it's in line with your body with the foot flexed. Using your stomach muscles, pull the leg back in and take it back out again.

2. Keep the movement controlled.

3. Do three sets of 15 repetitions on each leg.

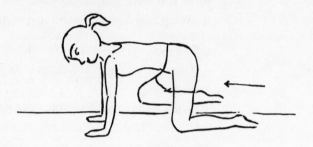

Hamstring curl on a Swiss ball:

These work your thighs, your bottom and your hamstrings.

1. Lie on your back with your legs straight and heels less than hip-width apart on a Swiss ball (giant blow-up ball – see Chapter 3).

2. Now lift your hips so that your body forms a straight line from your heels to your shoulders, and slowly bend your knees and

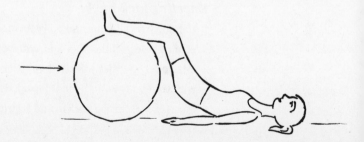

use your heels to pull the ball towards your bottom, and then roll back to the start position.

3. Do 15 repetitions.

Lunge walk:

This works your thighs, hamstrings and bottom and is perfect to do in your hallway.

1. Stand with your feet hip-width apart and take a step forwards. In the same movement lower your body down (as in a normal lunge), but don't let your front knee travel over your toe. Then rise up (by pushing through your heel) and step forwards with the other leg and repeat along the corridor.
2. Carry 6kg weights to make the exercise more challenging.
3. Do two sets per leg.

Saggy boobs and flabby, batwing arms

If your batwings and boobs jiggle more freely than they should – you're not alone, but you can wear a strappy top with pride by doing these exercises four times a week (fat burning is also essential for muscle definition, so make sure you do your cardiovascular session as well).

Lateral raise:

This helps tone and shape your shoulders and lats (the muscles under your armpits).

1. Stand up straight with your feet hip-width apart, shoulders

shoulders
+
under armpit
3×15

pulled down (imagine your shoulder blades sliding down your back) and stomach pulled in.

2. Now, holding 4kg weights in your hands at your sides and your elbows slightly bent, raise the weights out to the sides until your hands are level with your shoulders with your palms facing the floor. Hold for a second, lower and repeat.

3. Do three sets of 15 repetitions.

Press-up:

Perfect for instant toning of the chest and the arms.

1. Start by placing your hands directly under your shoulders (palms facing forwards). If you want to put more emphasis on the chest, place your arms wider; if you want to focus on the arms, place your hands closer in to your body.

2. Keeping your stomach pulled in and your body straight (or resting on your knees if you're a complete beginner), bend your arms to 90 degrees, then push yourself back up and start again. The trick is to pull down under your arms to support your body and support your back with your stomach muscles.

3. Build to three sets of 12 repetitions.

Triceps dip:

The triceps are the underused muscles on the underneath of your arm.

1. Sit on the edge of a sturdy chair, place your hands either side of your bottom and hold on to the edge of the chair. Your legs should be hip-width apart and bent to 90 degrees.

tip

Exercise without a healthy diet means slower results all round.

chest + arms

2. Start by moving your bottom forwards off the chair and then lower your bottom towards the floor by bending your arms, and then rise up by pushing up with your arms.

3. Do three sets of 10–15 repetitions. To make the exercise more challenging straighten your legs (move them further away from your body).

The triceps overhead:

triceps 4

1. Stand with your back straight. Find a weight that's challenging (i.e., it takes effort, not pain, to lift it) and hold it in one hand. Bending your arm, place the weight behind your head (your elbow should now be level with your head).

2. From this position lift the weight upwards, keeping your elbow close to your head, and lower slowly.

3. Do three sets of 15 repetitions on each arm.

Swiss ball triceps dip:

triceps + abs 5

This is an advanced exercise, which works on your stomach and arms so it pays to have a friend standing behind you just in case you feel unsafe.

1. Sit on top of a Swiss ball (the ball creates an unstable surface, which means you have to work your core stomach muscles to support you once you start the exercise) and place your hands either side of your bottom on the ball.

2. Your legs should be hip-width apart and bent to 90 degrees. Now move your bottom forwards off the ball and then lower it

towards the floor by bending your arms and then rise up by pushing up with your arms (the ball is meant to wobble).

3. Do two sets of ten repetitions.

The single arm row:

This works the biceps, backs of the shoulders and upper back.

-upper back
-biceps
-back of shoulders

1. Place your right hand and knee on a bench, and leave your left leg on the floor (in the correct position your back should now be as flat as a tabletop and parallel to the bench).
2. Now hold a weight in your left hand so that your arm hangs towards the floor. Pull the weight towards your chest in a rowing motion, but keep your shoulder still, and repeat.
3. Do three sets of 12 repetitions on each side.

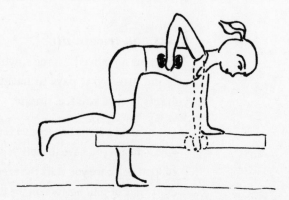

shoulders + Biceps

The upright row:

This is excellent for the shoulder muscles and biceps.

1. Stand with feet hip-width apart and back straight (shoulder blades pulled down). Hold weights (choose between 3–6kg) in front of your thighs (palms facing inwards).
2. From this position in a rowing motion lift the weights to chest height (leading with elbows) and return.
3. Do three sets of 15 repetitions.

Biceps curl:

For those sexy upper-arm-muscle bumps.

1. Stand up straight with your feet hip-width apart, shoulders back and stomach pulled in with your hands by your side.
2. Now, with your palms facing upwards, hold a 6kg (13¼lb) weight in each hand and lift it towards your chest and return to the start position. Be sure to keep your upper body still so you use your arm muscles to lift.
3. Do three sets of 10–15 repetitions.

Biceps

tip

Don't skip exercises you find hard. These are the ones you need to be doing.

Wobbly bellies

If you have a noticeable wobble it's worth noting that for a flatter stomach you have to combine tummy exercises with a low-fat diet or else your newly formed six-pack will be stuck under a layer of flab.

Lower abdominal raise:

1. Lie on your back with your knees bent, and lift your legs into the air at a 90-degree angle. Keep your arms by your side with your palms facing upwards.
2. Now pull your belly button to your spine and slowly lower one leg to the floor and bring it back up. This exercise is deceptively hard, so if you can't feel anything, you haven't pulled your stomach in or you're not lowering your leg slowly enough.
3. Do two sets of ten repetitions on each leg.

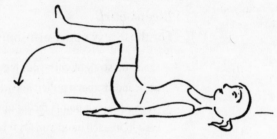

Army sit up:

1. Lie down on the floor with your knees bent. Place your feet together and anchor them under your sofa (though make sure your sofa's secure or else it will end up on your head).
2. Now loop a towel around the back of your neck and hold each end. Contract your tummy (keep your belly button pulled to your spine) and curl upwards, lifting your shoulders, head and back. Lower almost to the floor and repeat. Avoid yanking your head up with the towel by pulling down under your arms the whole time.
3. Do two sets of ten repetitions.

The hundreds:

1. Lie on the floor with your legs straight up in the air (if your back hurts, bend your knees as you keep your legs raised). Keep your arms at your sides but let them hover above the ground, palms facing down.
2. Contract your abdominals and lift your head, shoulders and upper body off the ground. In this position start to beat your arms up and down, slowly breathing in and then breathing out for a count of ten.
3. Repeat ten times and relax.

Upward bicycle:

1. Lie on the floor, and place your hands behind your head. Now bring your head and shoulders forward (use your stomach muscles, do not yank yourself forwards) and hold.
2. Lift your knees up to a 45-degree angle and start moving your legs in a bicycle motion. Do ten forward movements and then ten backward movements.
3. Rest and repeat three times.

Roll-up on a Swiss ball:

1. Sit up on the ball with your feet flat on the floor. Let the ball roll slowly back, and then slowly walk your feet forwards, and let your body slide down the ball until your thighs are parallel with the floor.
2. Your upper body should be resting on the ball. Hold yourself steady by pulling your stomach in (navel to spine). Now cross

your arms in front of your chest and lift your upper body forwards into a 'C' and return to start position.

1. Repeat ten times.

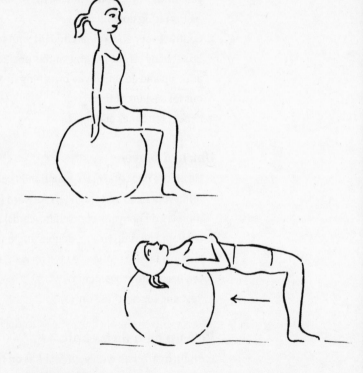

Ball reach:

1. Lie down flat on the floor with your thighs pressed firmly together. Hold a ball between your hands (a tennis ball will do) and raise your arms to the ceiling so the ball is above your chest.

2. Now, contracting your stomach and bottom, lift your shoulders

off the floor. Aim the ball upwards rather than forwards, lower, and repeat in a continuous movement.

3. Do two sets of ten repetitions.

Knee lift:

1. Sit on the edge of a sturdy chair with your knees bent and your feet flat on the floor. Hold on tight to the edge of the chair and tighten your stomach.
2. Lean back slightly and, keeping the knees bent and pressed together, lift your feet a few centimetres (inches) off the ground. Now slowly pull your knees upwards as you crunch your body forwards (not too far or else you'll fall off), lower feet and repeat.
3. Do two sets of ten.

The plank:

This works the deep layer of abdominal muscle known as the transversus abdominals.

1. Lie face down on the floor, and with elbows bent, clasp your hands together in front of your face and balancing on your forearms and toes, lift your body into a flat plank position. Your back should be flat, and your head aligned with your spine. Be

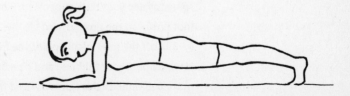

careful not to drop your bottom too far down, or lift it too high (do it in front of a mirror).

2. Hold this position for 10–15 seconds. Release to the floor and repeat three to five times.

Thunder thighs

Lovely lean thighs can be yours if you do these exercises three times a week.

Wide squat:

A wide squat is good for shaping your inner thighs and the front and back of the thigh.

Always combine shape-up exercises with cardio work for maximum results.

1. Stand with your feet wide apart and your toes turned out. Keeping your hands on your hips, lower your bottom towards the floor, as if you were about to sit down, keeping your upper body upright (pull that tummy in).

2. Go as low as you can without wobbling forwards, and then push back through your feet to the start position.

3. Do three sets of 15.

Leg circles:

1. Lie on your back on the floor, and pull your belly button to your spine to keep your back supported. Bend one knee, leaving the foot firmly on the ground, and lift the other leg about 13–20cm (5–8in) off the ground and point the foot.

2. Now, keeping your tailbone and hips firmly on the ground, make five small circles clockwise and five anticlockwise and

then change legs. Make sure the movement starts from the tops of your thighs (imagine your whole leg rotating).

3. Do three sets of 12 repetitions.

Inner thigh squeeze:

The perfect exercise for inner thighs.

1. Lie on your back with your legs bent and your feet on the floor. Now place a relatively firm cushion between your knees and hold it there.
2. Take a deep breath and, as you exhale, lift your hips off the ground while squeezing the cushion with your thighs for eight counts, and relaxing.
3. Keeping your hips up, repeat ten times.

Side-lying abduction (1):

This exercise works your outer thighs:

1. Lie on your side with your legs straight and in line with your hips and shoulders. Bend the knee beneath you for support (keep your back supported by pulling your stomach in) and lift your top leg as high as you can – imagine your leg being pulled from the heel.
2. Pause at the top, and then slowly bring the leg down and repeat.
3. Do two sets of 20 repetitions per leg.

Side-lying abduction (2):

This exercise works your inner thigh:

1. Lie on your side with your legs straight and in line with your hips and shoulders. Bend your top leg, and rest it in front of you on the floor.
2. Now raise and lower the underneath leg being sure to lift it from the top of the inner thigh.
3. Do two sets of 20 repetitions per leg.

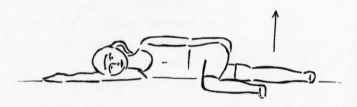

Side lift:

Excellent for working your outer thighs and whittling down your waist.

1. Lie on your left side, with your knees slightly bent towards your chest and your head resting on your left arm.
2. Raise your right leg and stretch it out, pushing through the heel. In this position, lift it 7.5cm (3in) (pull your tummy in), imagining your leg being pulled straight at all times. Repeat 15 times. Turn over and swap legs.
3. Do three sets of 15 repetitions.

Straight leg curl up:

This works your inner thighs, outer thighs and stomach.

1. Lie down on your back with your legs firmly pressed together and your toes pointed. Lift your arms over your head and breathe in.
2. Contracting your stomach and really squeezing your thighs together, bring your arms back over your head and curl your body up towards your feet. If you can't go all the way just lift your shoulders and head off the ground.
3. Breathe out and lower down (slowly), and repeat ten times.

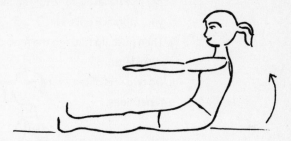

Inner thigh lift:

This tones the whole thigh area.

1. Lie backwards, resting on your elbows. Now bend your left leg and place the foot on the ground. Lift the right leg to the height of your left knee, once there rotate the leg out and lower to the floor.
2. Repeat 12 times on each leg.
3. Do three sets of 12 repetitions.

Totty pins

If you want to turn tree-trunk legs into luscious and lovely legs, here's how to do it.

Reverse lunge:

1. Stand 60–90cm (2–3ft) away from a chair with your back to it. Place your feet hip-width apart and put your hands on your hips for balance. Now, pulling in your stomach, rest the toes of one foot on the edge of the seat (your knee should be bent).

2. Slowly bend the other leg to 90 degrees (making sure the knee doesn't travel over the toe) and keeping your torso upright and your stomach pulled in.

3. Then push up through the foot, and repeat ten times and swap legs.

4. Do two sets of ten repetitions.

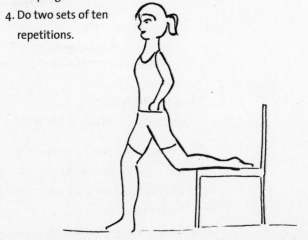

Static lunge:

This exercise works the inner thighs and bottom.

1. Take a large stride and place one foot in front of you (keep your hips pointing forwards) and your tummy pulled in.
2. Now bend your knees so your front leg drops forwards (don't let your knee travel over your toes) and your back leg drops down.
3. Push back through the heel of your foot to rise (this will work your bottom) and repeat.
4. Do two sets of 20 repetitions on each leg.

Squat with calf raise:

1. Stand with your feet slightly wider than hip-width apart (stomach in) and keep your hands at your sides. Squat down until your thighs are parallel to the floor, lifting your arms in front of you.
2. Move back to the starting position but extend past it and rise on to the balls of your feet, hold for one count and return to start position. Repeat the whole move.
3. Do two sets of 12 repetitions on each leg.

Plié with press back:

This is perfect for your calves, inner thighs, outer thighs and glutes (bottom).

1. Stand with your feet turned out at 45 degrees and slightly wider than shoulder-width apart.

tip

Stretch before and after all exercise to help your muscles lengthen as they strengthen.

2. Keep your knees soft (not locked) and bend your knees, until your thighs are parallel to the floor, raising your arms to chest height as you bend.
3. In this position, using your muscles, pull your inner thighs in and out four times and then, squeezing your bottom, return to standing.
4. Do two sets of 15 repetitions.

Lying kick:

This works the hips, bottom and legs.

1. Lie on your left side and bend your left leg beneath you and support your head with your left hand.
2. Now, pulling your stomach in, bring your right knee as close to your chest as you can (at hip height), flexing the foot. Slowly kick the leg out straight until it's fully extended through the heel. Keeping it at hip height bring it back to the start position.
3. Do two sets of ten repetitions on each leg.

Beats and paddles:

1. Lie face down on the floor, pulling in your stomach muscles and pushing your pubic bone to the floor.
2. Now lift your legs off the ground by about 5cm (2in) and beat your legs and heels together for a count of 50.
3. Relax, then go back into position and beat your feet up and down as if you were paddling in a small movement – again for 50 counts.

Step raise:

Perfect for perfect calves.

1. Using your upper-body weight for resistance and holding weights (4kg) in your hands, stand on a step with the balls of the feet on the step and heels hanging off the edge.
2. Lift your heels as high as you can (go on to the balls of your feet) and then lower your heels below the step's level to feel a stretch. If this feels too precarious, lift up on one leg as you lower the other, and repeat ten times on each leg.
3. Do two sets of ten repetitions.

Lunge kick:

Works the thighs and hamstrings.

1. Stand with your feet shoulder-width apart, and then step back into a lunge with your right leg. From the ground push back off the right foot. As you come back, transfer the weight to the left leg and kick the moving leg (right leg) slowly out in front of you, and then bring it back into a lunge and repeat.
2. Do two sets of ten repetitions on each leg.

20 ways to tone up

1 Work out your muscle hit list
It pays to buy an anatomy book (try the kids' section of your local bookstore) so you can workout where your gluteus medius is, from your gluteus minimus – that's your bottom by the way. Being muscle-aware will help you to target the areas you want to firm up.

2 Don't skimp on the cardio
It's tempting to give the run/walk/cycle a miss, but to lose weight effectively and tone up you need regular breathless exertion at least three times a week for at least 20 minutes.

3 Set attainable goals
Peach bottom in two weeks? Not unless you have plastic surgery, but a firmer bottom in six weeks can definitely be yours. Set goals that will spur you on, not have you reaching for the cream cakes.

4 Anchor your tongue
Basically, place your tongue on the roof of your mouth when you do a sit-up or any abdominal exercise. This stops your neck from aching by stabilising it, which, in turn, helps you to work your stomach and not get too tired too quickly.

5 Do compound exercises
These are exercises that work large and small muscle groups at the same time and both challenge your balance and activate your core muscles as you work. For example, doing weights on a Swiss ball, or standing on an unstable surface as you lunge.

6 Think navel to spine at all times
Even when you're at the bus stop, as this will immediately work your stomach, support your back and improve your posture, and it will make the move second nature when you're exercising.

7 Snack on foods your diet is short on
If you don't eat much dairy, have some cheese; a bag of mini carrots if

you're not getting your five servings of vegetables; a smoothie if you don't eat fruit; or almonds if you don't eat oily fish. This will keep your vitamin count high.

8 Eat before you exercise

Don't fool yourself that you'll burn more fat if you're hungry. The fact is that if you have no energy to burn because you haven't eaten you won't have the stamina to work out. Eat a light snack one hour before you work out.

9 Drink more to work out harder

Your body also craves more water; drink two glasses of water an hour before you exercise, and another one half an hour before. Throughout your workout drink before you're thirsty (thirst is a sign you're already dehydrated).

10 Mix up your routine

The body adapts quickly to an exercise routine, especially cardiovascular work, so be sure to either change your aerobic activity or keep challenging yourself. Try running, aqua jogging, power-walking, skipping, swimming, cycling and/or a dance class.

11 Get more active

Don't just use an exercise routine as an excuse to laze about even more. Every little thing helps; even washing your car for 30 minutes burns off 150 calories.

12 Don't forget your posture

For an instant posture improver, stand with the back of your head touching the wall. Keeping your body straight and feet flat on the floor (there should be a triangle shape between your body and the wall), hold this position for 60 seconds.

13 Count yourself in

To get maximum results from toning and lifting exercises, the key is slowness. Don't rely on momentum to get you from top to bottom, but count yourself in, breathing in for one count, lifting for one count, holding for one count and releasing.

14 Train your brain

Exercise studies show you can maximise your benefits by focusing your mind on the muscles you're working. Think of each muscle contracting and stretching as you move through the routine.

15 Listen to music

Studies from the Reebok University show that listening to music while you work out can push you to work harder. Stick to fast up-tempo dance CDs rather than heart-tugging tunes.

16 Don't forget to breathe

It sounds silly, but most of us forget to breathe when we're concentrating on something difficult. If you feel dizzy or light-headed after one move, the chances are you need to breathe more. Inhale to lift a weight, exhale to lower.

17 Know your limits

A heated burning feeling in your muscles shows that you're overworking the muscle to good effect, but a sharp pain means stop what you're doing now!

18 Don't rest too much

Never stop for more than a minute between exercises. Shorter recovery periods (where you try to get your breath back) means improved muscle endurance and better muscles all round.

19 Don't lift weights every day

This is over-training. Muscles need 48 hours to recover and repair. Meaning you'll get better results if you skip a day between strength-toning exercises.

20 If you're stiff and sore

Have a hot bath, to help soothe your aching limbs. If this happens a lot, you are not warming up and cooling down properly. You need to bring your heart level down with some gentle exercise for five minutes to aid the removal of lactic acid, the main contributor behind post-exercise soreness.

chapter 6
The bikini-fit six-week plan

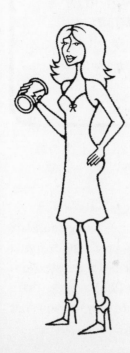

If you're a true lazy girl you probably shelved your good intentions to get in shape slowly months ago and are now facing your biggest challenge – a two-week beach holiday and no time to get in bikini shape. But before you throw yourself into starvation and over-exercising mode, give our six-week bikini-fit plan a try. It's tough, but if you do this you don't need to do the exercises in Chapters 3 and 4.

However, before you start the plan, bear in mind the following:

- This is not a crash diet, because a starve-yourself food plan (even for a fabulous event) will just cause your metabolism to slow down and cling on to every single thing you eat, making it harder for you to lose weight overall.
- The plan incorporates a fitness plan and an eating plan, both of which you have to do. This is because if you change your diet

but don't exercise you'll lose weight but you'll still look flabby. And if you exercise madly but live on chocolate and crisps, you'll be firmer but still appear the same size.

The bikini success equation is simple: eat less (or rather, eat more healthily) and do more (as in get off the sofa), and we guarantee you'll look fabulous in six weeks.

> ### The bikini-fit plan is the perfect plan for lazy girls because:
>
> - It lasts only six weeks.
> - It's so precise that all you have to do is follow it word for word.
> - It works!

The food rules

Follow the eating plan precisely, because eating chocolate bars instead of meals and/or skipping breakfast, or trying to lose half a stone in one week is a recipe for disaster. Aim to lose between 450g (1lb) and 900g (2lb) a week (that's over 6kg (1 stone) in six weeks), and not only will you do it but also the weight will stay off.

What you can do

- Eat unlimited amounts of vegetables and salad (but not potatoes) the greener and leafier the better. But don't fry them, add butter or drown them in olive oil and salad dressing. Try balsamic vinegar for salads and black pepper or soy sauce on stir-fried or steamed vegetables.

- Drink at least 2 litres (3½ pints) of water a day, and diet drinks, tea and coffee (with skimmed milk, skip the lattes and cappuccinos). Be careful of fruit juices, as they are loaded with sugar; if you can't resist them, dilute them with water.

- Always choose lean cuts of meat about the size of your palm. With chicken, take off the skin, and with red meat trim off the fat before cooking.

- Opt for wholemeal bread; anything made from white flour will just bloat you up and give you zero nutritional goodness.

- Think about how you cook and shop – don't fall into the olive oil and low-fat trap. Yes, olive oil is healthier than other oils, but it's still oil. Low fat doesn't mean low calorie or low sugar – scoff a whole bag of low-fat crisps, and you've nearly eaten the equivalent of a small meal in one go.

- Drink alcohol, but not too much, or else you'll end up drinking your calories. Indulging every day or binge drinking on week-ends (even if you don't eat) will ruin your chances of losing weight.

- Have a little bit of what you fancy. There are no good or bad foods, only bad eating habits.

- Think about what you drink; non-diet sodas carry as much as 8–13 teaspoons of sugar per can.
- Ideally you should drink 40 minutes before a meal, not during a meal, as water dilutes the digestive enzymes needed to break down your food, so that the food takes longer to digest.
- Don't multi-task and eat. If you eat too fast, or when you're stressed you won't chew food properly, and you'll end up washing your food down and swallowing too much air, which causes stomach bloating, wind and that tight waistband feeling.
- Add variety to all your meals. Too many of us eat cereal-sandwich-pasta every day, which equals a wheat overload, which in turn causes bloating.
- Avoid any food that ends in an '-ose' as it's basically a sugar. This will upset the bacterial balance in your stomach and cause bloating. Also avoid pre-packed processed meals, as they are loaded with chemicals, salt and sugar; all things that cause belly bloating and work against flat stomachs.
- Eat breakfast every day. The reason behind this thinking is simple: your body needs fuel in the morning. Not only has it not eaten for at least ten hours but also research shows that those who skip breakfast lack concentration at work, eat more at lunch and dinner, and snack more during the day because they haven't revved up their metabolism.
- Watch your portions, because if you can't be bothered to weigh your food the chances are you're eating too much. While you can eat as many vegetables (not potatoes) as you want, be

tip

If in doubt think raw, fresh and steamed – that way you know there are no hidden extras and no extra calories lurking below.

careful of fruit. As for portions of meat and fish – it's simple, never eat any piece that's bigger than the palm of your hand.

Sample menus

If you can't be bothered to think up your own menus, you can choose from the list below, which are all low fat and low calorie. If you're someone who buys all her meals ready-made, always check the labels for fat and sugar content before you buy. Try not to exceed 1,500 calories a day and make sure your fat levels don't exceed 50g (2oz) a day.

Breakfast options (one a day):

- Two pieces of rye bread with one teaspoon of peanut butter.
- One piece of fruit bread toasted, with a small tub of cottage cheese.
- 30g (1oz) of cooked oat porridge with skimmed milk and one teaspoon of honey or fresh, chopped fruit.
- Chopped apple, small bio yoghurt and two crispbreads.
- Two poached or boiled eggs on rye toast.
- One scrambled egg with a piece of wholemeal toast.
- 200g (7oz) baked beans (small can) on two pieces of toast.
- Two Weetabix with skimmed milk and a banana.
- One low-fat bran muffin and skimmed-milk cappuccino.
- A 30g (1oz) bowl of cereal with skimmed milk, and a small banana/apple.

Drink options (daily):

- Tea or coffee.
- A glass of fruit juice.
- A small glass of wine or a spirit measure with diet mixer.
- Diet colas.
- 2 litres (3½ pints) of water.
- 150ml (¼ pint) of skimmed milk.
- Herbal teas.

Snacks (have two of these a day):

- One tablespoon of hummus or 113g (3½oz or half a pot) cottage cheese on two oatcakes.
- Small serving of fruit – small banana, or apple.
- Cottage cheese with rice cakes.
- A small packet of unsalted nuts, preferably almonds.
- Yoghurt with a piece of fruit.
- A small pot (100g or 3½oz) of fromage frais and cut vegetables.
- A 25g (1oz) bar of chocolate.

Lunch (one a day):

- Pasta (the dried amount should fit into the palm of your hand) mixed with a small can of tuna or a teaspoon of pesto and a mixed salad with fruit.
- A jacket potato with dense vegetables (broccoli, cauliflower or cabbage) and a small serving of low-fat cheese (about half a pot).

- Buy a piece of ready-cooked chicken or fish (not smoked), a packet of mixed salad leaves, and ready-cut vegetables and mix together with balsamic vinegar.
- Tortilla wrap with chicken or a large salad and two boiled eggs or half a pot of cottage cheese. One tip to remember: always make sure your filling outweighs the wrap.
- Takeaway sushi, or buy two ready-made sandwiches and take the top layer off and eat as open sandwiches with a piece of fruit.
- Pitta and hummus – get two small, round pitta breads and put one tablespoon of hummus in each one and mix with raw vegetables.
- Tuna or egg bagel and an orange – slice and fill a bagel with egg or tuna and mix with a tablespoon of cottage cheese or low-fat soft cheese. Serve with a side salad.
- Small pitta bread with 185g (6½oz) of tuna in brine and salad.
- Granary roll with 50g (2oz) of reduced-fat Edam cheese and salad.
- Medium-sized jacket potato (no butter) with 80g (3oz) of tuna mixed with one boiled egg (or one egg and a small pot of cottage cheese).

Dinner (one a day):

- Grilled prawn, or chicken, or two eggs and cottage cheese salad (half a pot), with vegetables – all salads should have mixed salad leaves and at least seven different vegetables, including a small avocado.

tip

Read labels – this way you'll start to realise where all those extra calories are coming from.

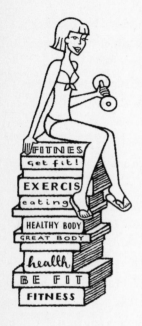

- Prawn and/or vegetable stir-fry – make sure you use a tiny bit of oil and flavour with herbs, and soy sauce. One piece of fruit.
- Steamed fish with broccoli and carrots, and a salad made up of mixed leaves, red peppers, tomatoes, avocado, cucumber and a teaspoon of pumpkin seeds.
- Grilled fish/chicken (no bigger than the size of the palm of your hand), oven-roasted peppers, mushrooms and courgettes, and a salad with fruit.
- Steamed or baked salmon on a bed of mixed leaves with avocado, tomatoes, peppers, green beans, mushrooms and carrots. A piece of fruit.
- Veggie curry – one medium potato, one onion, one diced pepper, one can of chopped tomatoes, cauliflower or spinach, chilli sauce and garlic. Before serving, add a small container of low-fat bio yoghurt (100g or 3½oz). Serve with four tablespoons of cooked rice.
- One large jacket potato and a small tin of baked beans plus three tablespoons of low-fat cheese with black pepper.
- 150g (5oz) of lean meat or Quorn with a vegetable stir-fry of broccoli, mushrooms, peppers and carrots, and a green side salad. For dressing the stir-fry and salad, opt for soy sauce, black pepper, chilli flakes and a teaspoon of honey.
- 100g (3½oz) of oily fish, such as salmon or mackerel, and watercress, spinach and bok choy vegetables, with a honey and soy-sauce dressing.

The fabulous exercise plan

Ten rules

1. Follow the instructions precisely.
2. Do not do more than three sessions a week, and only work out for one hour at the most.
3. Warm up and cool down for five minutes before exercising.
4. Always drink water throughout (or you'll pass out).
5. Eat at least one hour before you workout, for energy.
6. Stop if you feel a sharp pain (a dull pulling feeling is your muscle working), or sick and faint.
7. Always see a doctor before you start exercising if you have a lot of weight to lose and/or you have an injury.
8. Don't overdo it in the beginning – this is the number-one reason why people stop exercising.
9. Give yourself a day's break in-between each workout for your body to recover.
10. Wear the right workout gear – especially on your feet.

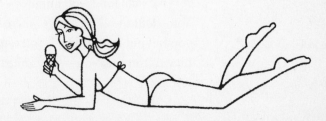

Props:

While this exercise plan has been designed for lazy girls who can't or won't get to a gym, there are a few props you'll need so that you can do this at home:

1. A Swiss ball (very cheap, see Resources).
2. Some weights (see Resources, or buy some tins of food in different sizes; bags of potatoes will do too).

Week 1 (three 45-minute sessions)

Warm up

Five minutes of aerobic exercise to gently raise your heartbeat (this gets oxygen to your muscles and gets you ready to work out). Try walking and then stretching.

Cardiovascular work

A brisk walk for 25–30 minutes – brisk as in nonstop walk. You should walk at a pace where breathing is difficult for you but not impossible. If you can talk but not have a fully blown conversation with someone, you're at the right intensity.

Toning

The standing lunge:

Good for your thighs and bottom.

1. Stand straight with your hands by your side, pull your stomach in (belly button to spine) and take one large step forwards, and, as the foot hits the ground, drop your body down, making sure your knee doesn't extend over your toes (don't lean forwards, and keep your body upright, and this won't happen).
2. Then spring back to starting position (it helps if you, push back with your front foot), and repeat.
3. Do ten repetitions per leg (five at a time) and do two sets (i.e., repeat the exercise twice).

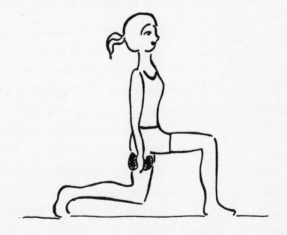

Press-up:

Good for chest muscles, flabby backs of arms and shoulder.

1. Start with a half press-up so your face doesn't smash into the floor. To do this, get on to your hands and knees and place your arms directly under your shoulders, keeping your hands pointing forwards.
2. Slowly lower the body to the ground and then lift up into the start position (it helps if you pull down under your arms as you push up).
3. Do two sets of ten repetitions.

Lateral raise:

Good for your shoulders and arms.

1. Grab two tins of beans – or 3kg weights – and sit down in a straight-backed chair. With your feet hip-width apart and your stomach pulled in, start with your arms by your side and with your hands facing towards your body.
2. Now, keeping your body still, slowly raise your arms away from your sides (keeping elbows unlocked) level with your shoulders, and then lower.
3. Repeat (do it slowly so your muscles work and you don't rely on momentum).
4. Do two sets of ten repetitions.

Abdominal crunch with twist:

Good for your waist and stomach.

1. Lie on your back with your knees bent, feet on the floor and your hands behind your head. Make sure there is a natural curve in your spine, your belly button is pulling towards your spine and your tailbone is down throughout.
2. Now, without yanking your head, but by using your stomach muscles, lift your upper body off the ground and twist your shoulder and elbow towards your opposite thigh. Change sides and repeat.
3. Do two sets of 20 repetitions.

tip

2-litre water bottles can also be used as handy home weights.

Week 2 (three 45-minute sessions)

Warm up

Five minutes of aerobic exercise to gently raise your heart-beat.

Cardiovascular work

1. Walk for four minutes, and then run for two minutes and repeat three times (18 minutes in total).
2. Then run for two minutes, walk for two minutes. Repeat three times (12 minutes in total). Total 30 minutes.

Toning

Step-up:

Works your calves, hamstrings and thighs. Do this exercise at a pace to raise your heartbeat.

1. Place one leg on a step, and keep the other on the floor. Now, with weights (3kg) in your hands, step up, lifting the back leg into the air in front of you, and then returning it to the start position.
2. Do two sets of 15 repetitions.

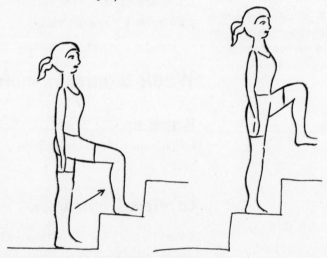

The standing lunge (see week 1):
Do two sets of 15 repetitions per leg.

One arm bent over row:
Works your arms, lats and biceps.

1. Rest your left hand and knee on a sturdy, flat coffee table (or put two chairs together), keeping your right foot on the floor. Hold a 3kg weight (or can of beans) in your right hand and let your arm hang towards the floor. Your back should be parallel to the table.
2. Now pull the weight towards your chest, keep your body stable, back straight and return to the start position. Make the movement slow and controlled (and focus on your back muscles).
3. Do two sets of 15 repetitions on each arm.

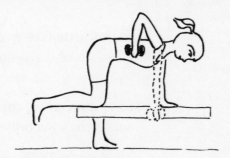

Press-up (three-quarter press-up):

1. This time get on to your hands and knees, and move forwards on your arms so that your knees are still on the floor but your body is stretched out.
2. Place your arms directly under your shoulders and slowly lower the body to the ground and then lift up into the start position.
3. Do two sets of 15 repetitions.

Shoulder press:

Works your shoulders and arms.

1. Sit down in a chair and, holding a 4kg weight in each hand, lift your arms out to the sides so that they are level with your shoulders. Bend your elbows (the weights should be level with the top of your head).
2. From this position press (as in push) the weight upwards, so that your arms are above your head (don't let your shoulders rise with your arms).
3. Do two sets of 15 repetitions.

tip

Aim to increase weights once exercises feel too easy.

Lateral raise (see week 1):

Do two sets of 15 repetitions.

Lower abdominal raise:

Tones flabby lower bellies.

1. Lie on your back with your knees bent, and lift your legs into the air at a 90-degree angle. Keep your arms by your sides with your palms facing upwards.
2. Now pull your belly button to your spine and keep it there throughout (don't pull it so tightly that you can't breathe), and slowly lower one leg to the floor and bring it back up. This exercise is deceptively hard, so if you can't feel anything, you

haven't pulled your stomach in or you're not lowering your leg slowly enough.

3. Do two sets of ten repetitions on each leg.

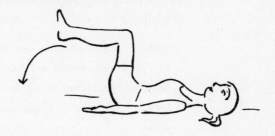

Abdominal crunch with a twist (see week 1):
Do two sets of 15 repetitions.

Week 3 *(three one-hour sessions)*

Warm up

Five minutes of aerobic exercise to gently raise your heartbeat.

Cardiovascular work

1. Run for three minutes, walk for two minutes and repeat three times (for 15 minutes).

2. Then run for four minutes and walk for one minute and repeat three times (for 15 minutes). Total 30 minutes.

Toning

Static lunge:

Works inner thighs and bottom (hold 4kg weights to make it harder).

1. Take a large step and place one foot in front of you (keep your hips pointing forwards) and your tummy pulled in.
2. Now bend your knees so your front leg drops forwards (don't let your knee travel over your toes) and your back leg drops down.
3. Push back through the heel of your foot to rise (this will work your bottom), and repeat.
4. Do two sets of 20 repetitions.

Step-up (see week 2):

Place some 4kg weights in your hands to make the exercise harder. Do two sets of 20 repetitions per leg.

Side-lying abduction (1):

Works your outer thighs.

1. Lie on your side with your legs straight and in line with your hips and shoulders. Bend the knee beneath you for support (keep your back supported by pulling your stomach in) and lift your top leg as high as you can – imagine your leg being pulled from the heel.
2. Pause at the top, slowly bring the leg down, and repeat.
3. Do two sets of 20 repetitions per leg.

Side-lying abduction (2):

Works your inner thighs.

1. Lie on your side with your legs straight and in line with hips
   and shoulders. Bend your top leg, and rest it in front of you on
   the ground. Now raise and lower the underneath leg being sure
   to lift it from the top of the inner thigh.
2. Do two sets of 20 repetitions on each leg.

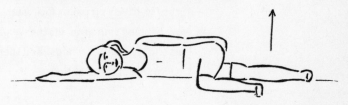

One arm bent over row (see week 2):

Lift heavier weights to increase the challenge. Do two sets
of 20 repetitions per arm.

Lying chest press:

Works flabby underarms and chest.

1. Lie facing upwards on a sturdy bench (make sure it can support
   your weight otherwise skip this one). Hold two weights in your
   hands above your chest (arms straight, palms facing forwards).
   Lower the weights towards your chest letting your elbows go
   past your body.
2. Do two sets of 20 repetitions.

Shoulder press (see week 2):

Do two sets of 20 repetitions.

Biceps curl:

Gives you killer arms.

1. Stand hip-width apart, with your stomach pulled in. Hold 4kg weights by your side in each hand, and, with your elbows tucked in, have your palms facing upwards.
2. Now, bending your arms, lift the weights towards your shoulders (curl your arm upwards), and then lower.
3. Do two sets of 20 repetitions.

Reverse curl:

Works the lower stomach muscles.

1. Lie on the floor with your legs in the air (keep your knees bent slightly) and your arms by your side, palms facing upwards.
2. Now, tightening your lower abdominals, lift your legs into the air and towards your ribs, hold for a second and then lower, and repeat.
3. Do two sets of 20 repetitions.

Lower abdominal raise (see week 2):

Do two sets of ten repetitions.

tip

With arm exercises don't let your shoulders do the work your arms should be doing. (Help yourself by consciously pulling your shoulders down.)

Week 4 *(three one-hour sessions)*

Warm up

Five minutes of aerobic exercise to gently raise your heart-beat.

Cardiovascular work

Run for eight minutes, walk for two minutes and repeat three times. Total time 30 minutes.

Toning

Lunge walk:

This works your thighs, hamstrings and bottom, and is perfect to do in your hallway.

1. Stand with your feet hip-width apart and take a step forwards. In the same movement, lower your body down (as in a normal lunge), but don't let your front knee travel over your toe.
2. Then rise up (by pushing through your heel) and step forwards with the other leg, and repeat along the corridor.
3. Do two sets of ten steps. Carry 6kg weights to make the exercise more challenging.

Squat:

Thighs, hamstrings and bottom.

1. Stand up straight and pull your stomach in and, holding 6kg weights at your side, bend your knees and squat down (as if

you were going to sit down). Your feet should stay flat and your body and legs shouldn't wobble.
2. Return to standing, and repeat.
3. Do two sets of 20 repetitions.

Step-up (see week 2):
Speed the pace up. Do two sets of 20 repetitions.

Side-lying abduction (1) and (2) (see week 3):
Do two sets of 20 repetitions.

Static lunge (see week 3):
Hold weights in each hand, go heavier to challenge yourself – 7kg. Do two sets of 20 repetitions.

One arm bent over row (see week 2):
Lift heavier weights – 8kg or two cans tied together. Do two sets of 20 repetitions.

Full press-up:
Works the arms and the chest.

1. Place your hands shoulder-width apart and keep your body and legs straight out behind you so that your body is in a perfect line (pull your stomach in to stop your back sagging).
2. Now slowly lower your body to the floor and push yourself back up to the start position, and lower again.
3. Do two sets of 20 repetitions.

Swiss ball shoulder press:
For shoulders, stomach and arms:

1. Holding 5kg weights (or heavy tins) in your hands, sit on the Swiss ball and bring your elbows to shoulder height.
2. Press the weights upwards and bring them back down. The unstable surface of the ball means you have to work your stomach hard to maintain stability as you lift the weights.
3. Do two sets of 20 repetitions.

Triceps dip:
Works your arms and triceps.

1. Facing away from a sturdy chair, place your hands on the edge of it and, keeping your feet hip-width apart, bend your knees, so your back and arms are straight.
2. In this position lower yourself down (keeping your bottom pushed back) until your elbows are bent, and then push back up until your arms are straight again.
3. Do two sets of 20 repetitions.

Biceps curl (see week 3):
Do two sets of 20 repetitions.

Lower abdominal raise (see week 2):
But this time lower and lift both legs at the same time in a controlled manner. Do two sets of 15 repetitions.

Abdominal crunch with twist (see week 1):
Do two sets of 20 repetitions.

Week 5 *(three one-hour sessions)*

Warm up
Five minutes of aerobic exercise to gently raise your heart-beat.

Cardiovascular work
Run for ten minutes, walk for one minute, and repeat three times. Total 33 minutes.

Toning
Swiss ball squat:
Works your thighs and bottom.

1. Place the Swiss ball between your middle back and a wall, and hold 5kg (11lb) weights in each hand.
2. From a standing position, drop down slowly into a squat until your thighs are parallel to the ground and then slowly push yourself up.
3. Do three sets of ten repetitions.

Lunge with two bounces:
This works your thighs and bottom.

1. Do a lunge as before (see week 1, standing lunge), but this time

when you drop down do two bounces to work the thigh. Rise back up and repeat.

2. Do three sets of 20 – if it's too easy, hold 6kg weights as you lunge.

Step-up (see week 2):

Up the pace, hold 7kg weights in each hand. Do three sets of 20 repetitions per leg.

Hamstring curl on a Swiss ball:

These work your thighs, your bottom and your hamstrings.

1. Lie on your back with your legs straight and heels less than hip-width apart on a Swiss ball.

2. Now lift your hips so that your body forms a straight line from your heels to your shoulders, and slowly bend your knees and use your heels to pull the ball towards your bottom. Then roll back to the start position.

3. Do three sets of 20 repetitions.

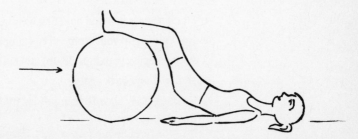

Side-lying abduction (1) and (2) (see week 3):
Do three sets of 20 repetitions.

One arm bent over row (see week 2):
Do three sets of 20 repetitions.

Lying chest press (see week 3):
Do three sets of ten repetitions.

Shoulder press (see week 2):
Do three sets of ten repetitions.

Lateral raise (see week 1):
Use 4kg weights. Do three sets of ten repetitions.

Triceps dip (see week 4):
Do three sets of 20 repetitions.

Biceps curl on a Swiss ball:
Front of arms

1. Sit on a Swiss ball and hold 6kg weights in your hands.
2. Now, pulling in your stomach to support you, lift one leg off the floor (keeping your hips down) and curl the weights to your shoulder and back again.
3. Do one set of ten with your left leg off the floor and swap legs for another set of ten.

Roll-up on a Swiss ball:

1. Sit up on the ball with your feet flat on the floor. Let the ball roll slowly back, and then slowly walk your feet forwards. Let your body slide down the ball until your thighs are parallel with the floor.
2. Your upper body should be resting on the ball. Hold yourself steady by pulling your stomach in (navel to spine). Now cross your arms in front of your chest and lift your upper body forwards into a 'C' and return to the start position.
3. Do two sets of 20 repetitions.

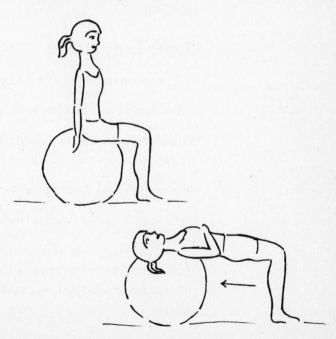

Week 6 *(three one-hour sessions)*

This final week is a circuit, which brings a cardiovascular edge to your workout. Both circuits should be repeated three times, with 90-second rests between circuits, not exercises. Clue: you should be shattered by the time you've done this.

Warm up

Five minutes of aerobic exercise to gently raise your heartbeat.

Upper-body circuit

Full press-up (see week 4): for 45 seconds.

Roll-up on a Swiss ball (see week 5): for 45 seconds.

Shoulder press with 5kg weights (see week 2): for 45 seconds.

Step-up (see week 2): at a pace, for 45 seconds.

Biceps curl with 5kg weights (see week 5): for 45 seconds.

Shuttle runs: place two markers 10m (33ft) apart in your garden or local park and run between them, for 45 seconds.

Lower abdominal lift (see week 2): lowering and lifting one leg at a time for 45 seconds.

Lateral raise with 5kg weights (see week 2): for 45 seconds.

Lower-body circuit

Swiss ball squat (see week 5): with 6kg weights in your hand, for 45 seconds.

Shuttle runs (see above): for 45 seconds.

Abdominal crunch with twist (see week 1): for 45 seconds.

Step-up: for 45 seconds.

Full press-up: for 45 seconds.

The standing lunge (see week 1): for 45 seconds.

Jog on the spot: for 45 seconds.

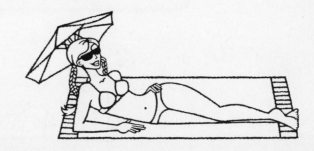

Lose weight without trying

If you:	You'll burn/save in a month:
Jump off the bus a stop earlier	600–1,000 calories
Climb some stairs every day	1,400 calories
Clean your kitchen (weekly)	400 calories
Walk over to a work friend instead of email	380 calories
Walk to the shops	600–700 calories
Swim for one hour a week	2,000 calories
Cycle for one hour a week	2,000 calories
Walk for one hour three times a week	3,600 calories
Wash your car once a week	1,120 calories
Mow the lawn once a week	1,600 calories
Sex (you on top) three times a week	1,800 calories
Sex (missionary)	960 calories
If you skip your daily chocolate bar you'll save	4,750 calories *a week*.

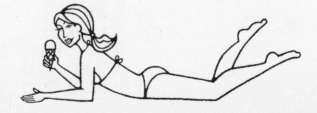

Oops ... you've slipped up!

If you've	Your payback is ...
Drunk two bottles of wine	To run an extra mile a day for a week (or walk two miles a day)
You've eaten a family-sized bag of sweets at the cinema	To cycle for half an hour every day for a week
Eaten a packet of crisps	To power-walk to work every day (one mile at least)
Drunk a latte a day	To climb stairs at a pace for five minutes, three times a week.
Eaten a chocolate croissant for breakfast	To swim three times a week

20 ways to stick to the plan

1 Anticipate potential problems
If you're about to start a new job, or are going through something stressful, or know you're away at weekends, work out how you're going to keep to the six-week plan before you start. Anticipating hurdles in advance means you'll deal with them more effectively.

2 Stop before you eat
If in doubt about what you're going to eat, ask yourself three questions: is this healthy? How hungry am I? And – will this sabotage my fabulous plan?

3 Think about your muscles
Studies show that focusing your attention on the muscle you're working helps build strength. Likewise think about how your running/cycling/swimming will improve your form and help you last longer.

4 Build a support team
Think of yourself like a racing driver, so when you make pit stops you have a support team on hand to encourage you, help you out and keep you motivated. Even better, do the plan with a friend to make sure neither of you cheat.

5 Think about solutions, not problems
It's easy when you start a plan to think of all the reasons it won't work, such as you have to work long hours/are on shift patterns/or are always tired. To succeed, focus on solutions, such as getting up earlier and working out in your lunch hour or before you come home. Better still, utilise your weekends.

6 Identify your weak areas
What time of day do you always think about breaking your healthy-eating plan or throwing away your exercise gear? If it's late afternoon and evening, do all your hard work in the morning to avoid flaking out. Likewise have ready-made snacks on hand to combat your need for sugary food.

7 Persevere

OK, let's be honest, you're going to feel horrible for the first few days, partly because this is a detox to your normal life, and partly because change is hard on your body. Yet studies show it just takes two days to start forming a new habit, which means by day three you'll be well on the way to looking fabulous.

8 Don't skip meals

You may think you're saving calories, but the truth is you'll only get them somewhere else. Also you won't do yourself any favours on the exercise front. To work out, you need energy, and for energy you need to eat at least three to four times a day.

9 Stay motivated

If you still aren't particularly inspired to move your butt, do something that will motivate you in your hardest hours. Buy an expensive bikini and keep it hanging in your bedroom on view (or by the fridge) to spur you on. Place last year's beach pics on your mirror to remind you of the new you, or promise yourself two weeks away when you reach your goal.

10 Stick to one plan at a time

So one friend's doing the eat-no-carbs diet, another is detoxing and yet another has a completely different exercise plan – don't compare and contrast. There are a million ways to lose weight and get fit, and if you mix and match you'll end up confused and unsure of where you're heading and why.

11 Do something about your stress levels

If you're stressed, you're at a higher than average risk of depression, and therefore less likely to stick to any plan, so don't make the plan yet another stress in your life. Instead prepare for the plan by clearing time in the next two weeks when you can start it effectively without having to worry about work/relationships/family or social events.

12 Tell yourself you can do it

If you don't believe you can do it, you won't be able to focus on the end result, and without a clear picture you won't be able to see an end result. Meaning, visualise the new you and keep that picture in your head as you're exercising and moving towards your goal.

13 Cut down on the booze

It's someone's birthday, you've got a new boyfriend, you're single, you're depressed, you've just worked out, oh, any old excuse for a quick one down the pub. Think like this and you'll not only sabotage your eating plan but also you won't be able to stir yourself into action for your fitness workouts. Put the booze on hold – it's only for six weeks, even you can do that!

14 Don't overdo it

It's great that you're so eager to get fit, but be wary of overdoing it. Be too zealous with your diet and workouts and you'll not only burn out fast but also place yourself at risk of injury (because your bones and muscles won't have time to recover in-between workouts and so be weaker when you use them).

15 Beware of weekend splurging

If you're sticking to the 1,500 calories a day on weekdays and then living it up on 2,500 a day (or more) at weekends, you're averaging up to 1,800 calories or more a day, meaning slower weight loss all round.

16 Don't have a fantasy goal

Goals are important, but pinning your hopes on getting an ideal body in six weeks if you're very unfit is a recipe for disaster. The goal is to look fabulous in six weeks – that's fitter, more toned, and trimmer than you are now, not transform yourself into a supermodel.

17 Work out at the right intensity

A new study shows 88 per cent of Americans think they exercise at the right intensity but less than 35 per cent actually do. You should be sweating, breathless and find the workout challenging (not soul destroying) – any less than that and you need to up the pace.

18 Eat more

If you feel faint, lacking in energy or sick (especially when you're working out) the chances are you're not eating enough. Don't be too rigid with portions and meals. If you feel hungry (measure it on a scale of one to ten) don't be afraid to add something to your diet.

19 Avoid comparing yourself to others

Don't put yourself under pressure by constantly comparing your body and your progress to others (both in the gym and on the street). It's a guaranteed way to give up.

20 Fall in love

This tactic works better than anything. Apart from causing an adrenaline surge that boosts your metabolic rate, it helps you lose your appetite and get down the gym like no other motivator.

chapter 7
A cheat's way to a fabulous body

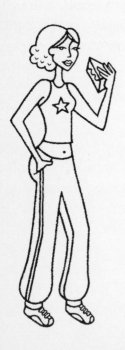

OK, so you've sweated it out, survived on vegetables and lean chicken, lifted weights until your biceps were as hard as walnuts, but still your fabulous body is a dream. Well, let's be honest here, the chances are you didn't do all of the above (or did it half-heartedly). If so, you'll be glad to know this chapter is dedicated to the laziest of the lazy. This is the place where we can shoehorn you into a bikini made of the strongest Lycra and help you troubleshoot your way into looking and feeling fabulous.

First up, there are many ways to cheat your way into a fabulous body, but most of these require lots of money, painful surgery and torturous underwear – think 18-hour girdles, tummy tucks and liposuction. Thankfully, there are also some good no-effort techniques for those days when you just have to look smaller and firmer.

Get some body confidence

Believe it or not, you can look fabulous without losing weight, exercising or squeezing yourself into a size ten pair of jeans, and all it takes is a change of attitude. The simple fact is true that confidence isn't about looks, or money, or the size of your breasts, it's simply about liking yourself, lumps, bumps, warts and all. Life shows us that size isn't everything, and if you don't believe me look around at all the people who aren't a perfect ten who are perfectly happy, perfectly in love, perfectly beautiful, clever, amusing and perfectly fabulous in their own right. If you're self-esteem is flagging, no amount of exercise plans and weight loss are ever going to make you feel good about yourself. To boost your self esteem:

tip

Get some body confidence and you'll be laughing while everyone else is too busy measuring themselves up in front of the mirror.

Change the record

Listing all the things wrong with you is a bit like hitting yourself over the head every day with a rolling pin. Don't victimise yourself. You don't have to be a certain size, weight, or height to be happy and look good.

Don't blame your parents

If you had an overtly critical parent who was always adept at crushing your confidence it can be easy to keep blaming them for how you feel. If this sounds familiar, bring yourself into the here and now and focus only on how you feel about yourself.

Sing your praises

You're not going to feel fabulous overnight, but if you start working on yourself you can start to feel better by tomorrow. Tell yourself your good points, highlight what's fantastic about you and remind yourself of the compliments people give you.

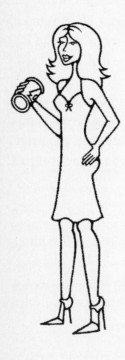

Accept compliments

Don't be someone who throws compliments back at their friends with lines such as, 'Oh no I'm not' or 'Oh, you're only saying that'. Tell people you're unattractive or fat and hate compliments enough and they'll stop sending them your way. Then be someone who compliments others – this is a sign of having good self-esteem and being able to think about someone other than yourself.

Be outward looking

Often people who feel bad about themselves spend too much time thinking about themselves. Think outwardly, and you'll be less concerned with your thighs/arms/flabby tummy.

Don't compare yourself to others

Do this and you run the risk of either feeling smug or horrible about yourself. It's a waste of time on another level, too, because no one has the same biological make up as you, meaning you're unique – so act that way.

Think about your body language

How you hold yourself makes more of an impact than you might think. Sit slumped over, and people won't notice you (well not in the way you want). Sit upright with your stomach pulled in and you'll appear more attractive than you ever thought possible.

Boost your metabolism

This is the truly sneaky way to lose pounds and burn more calories than your friends do. Contrary to popular belief, over 60 per cent of your daily calories are not burnt through that 30-minute jog you just did around the park but by what's known as your resting metabolic rate (the rate your body uses up energy when you're basically lounging about doing nothing). And this rate is influenced by a number of factors that you can influence:

Exercise: you can boost your metabolic rate with exercise. Especially if you increase the amount of lean muscle you have, as muscles need more calories to function than body fat does.

How hard you work out: the more intense your workout, then the longer your metabolism will be boosted.

How healthy your eating habits are: low-calorie diets lower your metabolism, simply because your body switches itself on to starvation mode and starts clinging on to everything you eat.

How much you eat: you can eat more than you think. Opt for six small, healthy meals a day, because every time you eat your metabolic rate goes up.

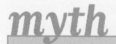

You're overweight because you have a slow metabolism. Untrue. Bigger people have high, not low, metabolisms because heavier bodies need more energy in order to function. But bigger people don't lose weight, because they eat more calories than they burn off.

Think positively

This is not an invitation to stand in front of the mirror and chant positive affirmations about how gorgeous you are (though if it helps, by all means do so). Being positive is about turning your weaknesses into strengths and being upbeat about who you are right now, not who you could be in a year's time. Easier said than done if, in your opinion, you're 100 miles away from being fabulous. However, the answer lies not in lying to yourself or pretending you're OK when you're not, but in finding practical solutions to help you look better, feel better and look your absolute best.

Solution 1: invest in some clothes that do your figure justice

Women are notorious at hiding their lumps and bumps under baggy T-shirts and unattractive sweatpants. Help yourself look good by accentuating your curves, by buying clothes that fit properly. Think fitted, not overly tight, and figure flattering, not the latest fashion.

Big boobs? Then think of a V-neck.

Fat tummy? Then think of a top that fits but also ripples along your waist.

Fat arms? Then think of sleeves that flute at the end.

Big bottom? Then think of tailored trousers and bootleg jeans.

Solution 2: buy the right underwear

Seventy-five per cent of us wear the wrong bra size. This includes you, if:

- You have rack marks across your skin when you take your bra off.
- Your breasts spillith over or under your bra cups.
- Your straps constantly fall down.

- The centrepiece of your bra doesn't lie flat across your ribcage.
- And you have no uplift whatsoever.

Solution 3: hold your head high

It's the old posture tip again. Hold your head up high (shoulders back, chest in, stomach in – imaginary piece of string pulling you up from the centre of your head) and you'll look lighter, appear more confident and pretty much get away with any look you want. Hunching, slumping and generally sitting curled up like a pretzel doesn't scream 'fabulous' to anyone.

To help keep your body flexible and bendy, you need to make sure you bend properly when lifting something. This means picking your undies off the floor while tottering around in high heels is a big no-no. The way to do it right is to maintain a straight back and then bend your knees as you go down and slowly rise to your original position.

Solution 4: sleep right

A rock-hard bed or soft mattress is not the best bet for a fabulous body. You need a mattress that will support the spine and allow it to stay in its natural curve as you move (i.e., the mattress should give as you move). If you can't afford a new mattress, department stores often sell mattress pads to help soften up a night's sleep. Above all, don't sleep on an old sagging mattress – experts recommend that a mattress be replaced every eight years.

Solution 5: sleep more

Good, healthy sleep is seven to eight hours a night, every night. It's about waking up feeling full of energy and not falling asleep on the bus into work. If you look and feel tired, you'll never feel fabulous no matter how much effort you put into exercise and diet. This is because our bodies need to sleep to boost our energy levels after being awake for 16–17 hours. For one whole week sleep for eight hours every night and observe the difference in your skin and your energy levels.

Solution 6: think about your lifestyle

High heels, smoking, drinking too much, eating kebabs at 1.0 a.m. and relying on caffeine to wake you up every day will all work against any exercise and healthy eating plan. If anything, it will simply cancel the other out leaving you in exactly the same place when you started this book. Meaning, if you want to feel better instantly, tone down your lazy girl ways (at least for the summer).

tip

When doing domestic-goddess chores, always keep upright and hold your stomach in to support you. If you feel curled over like a pretzel, stand up, stretch and roll your shoulders backwards and forwards until they warm up.

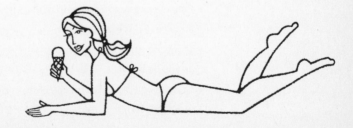

Try a lazy weekend detox

Even the laziest girl in the world can manage a healthy weekend (especially if you get your friends to hide your money and take away all the tempting food and alcohol in your house first). Detoxing is a spring-clean system where you limit your diet for a short period of time, in order to kick-start your body.

The detox rules

- Turn off your phone, get a pile of videos, magazines and CDs, and then tell your friends you're going away for the weekend.
- Clear the sofa (you'll need it to lie on), spring-clean your house, so you won't be tempted to do it while you're detoxing.
- Get in all the food you'll need for the detox the day before and then either lock away all tempting food, or give it to your friends.
- Prepare raw veggies, cut up fruit in advance so you won't have an excuse not to eat it.
- Stockpile some beauty products so you can slap on a face mask as you lie on the sofa detoxing.
- Grab a yoga or Pilates video – who knows, you might feel in the mood to stretch at some point (or see Chapter 3).

- When you start to detox, remember to take things easy, as you'll begin to feel tired when the process starts to work.
- Drink lots of water all weekend – at least 2 litres (3½ pints) a day – to stop dehydration and to speed up the cleansing and reviving process.
- Open a window – detoxing can be a stinky process.
- Finally, never detox if you are pregnant, breastfeeding, on medication, are diabetic, have kidney or liver problems, or are ill.

myth

Detoxes are scary. Unlike the scary regimes of the past, these days a detox diet doesn't mean fasting for days. In fact, starving yourself can actually be harmful to the body as it releases too many toxins too quickly and can leave you feeling dizzy, plus giving you headaches, bad breath and terrible skin.

What not to eat

If you want to revive your skin and energy levels, try this lazy girl detox. As the main aim of detoxing is to cleanse your body, you need to do two things: (1) help encourage the removal of toxins, and (2) limit your intake of new toxins.

To limit new toxins, cut out:

- Coffee and tea. Five cups a day can lead to caffeine toxicity, which results in restlessness, dry skin and tiredness.

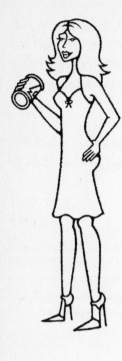

- Alcohol. This is super-toxic and can lead to liver damage, heart strain and dehydration.
- Salt. This definitely needs to be eliminated during a detox, as it aids dehydration and causes bloating.
- Sugar. Again, it's essential to avoid sugar (in the form of chocolate and cakes) during a detox, because it accelerates mood swings and headaches.
- Dairy. Believed to be mucus-forming foods, which release toxins that cause sinus problems and skin complaints.

What to eat

Instead eat:

- Lean meat and fish.
- Fruit and green, leafy vegetables.
- Opt for wholegrain produce.
- Drink lots of water.

Day 1

Start the day with a glass of warm water and lemon juice to flush out your system.

Breakfast

Eat fruit: grapes, apples and melon are a good choice, rather than bananas, which tend to be too starchy. Add a tablespoon of plain, live bio yoghurt. For a drink, make yourself a pot of herbal tea.

Fruit is an excellent start to the day, as it helps to activate the liver (the body's main cleansing organ) and stimulate the bowel, and it still gives you all the essential vitamins and minerals you need. The live bio yoghurt will help to cleanse and balance up the good and bad bacteria in your gut.

Lunch
Make a salad with as much mixed raw vegetables as you want. Use a teaspoon of olive oil on the salad and a piece of steamed fish or tofu.

The enzymes in the raw vegetables will boost your metabolism and give you some much-needed energy, while the fibre will speed up the cleansing process.

Snacks
Hungry? Then snack on grated carrots or apple slices, and/or drink plenty of water.

Dinner
Aim to have your last meal of the day before 8.0 p.m., as this gives you plenty of time to digest the food before going to sleep. Though raw is best, if you can't face another salad, lightly steam some fresh vegetables, or stir-fry them in a wok with tofu or lean meat, and season to taste.

Days 2 and 3
Stick to the above diet, but add a jacket potato, and/or some short-grain brown rice to your steamed vegetables at dinner and your salad at lunch.

tip

Don't detox when you have PMS – your body needs more energy prior to your period.

Extras

Enhance your detox by taking care of your skin. It's one of the biggest organs of toxin elimination, and skin brushing will help stimulate the lymphatic system to get the toxins moving towards the surface of the skin.

For a face pack on the cheap, go for mashed banana and honey. For a body scrub, porridge oats, massage oil and a ripe avocado. To come out smelling sweetly, place drops of lavender and jasmine oil under the bath tap to scent your skin and infuse your place with cleansing smells.

Ten ways to make the detox last

1. Eat five servings of fruit and vegetables a day.
2. Drink at least 8–12 glasses of water a day.
3. Cut down on coffee.
4. Eat lean meats and fish.
5. Learn to relax and de-stress.
6. Don't eat late at night.
7. Take an antioxidant supplement. This will help fight off daily pollutants that attack the body.
8. Stop smoking – the perfect way to stop toxins entering your body.
9. Drink less.
10. Sleep eight hours a night.

Treat yourself

Looking good is also about having a body that feels good. If the thought of having someone lavish endless attention on your body with beauty products makes you sigh with pleasure, then you'll know what I mean. However, if you're tired, and have skin, hair and nails that would make a cave woman proud, it's unlikely you've got to grips with the art of body therapies. Give the following a try – they'll make you look and feel better than you think:

Body wraps

Think beauty-salon treatments, especially Thalgo, Decleor and Guinot. Most body wraps, whether they are hot or cold, work on a firming, exfoliating and trussing-you-up-in-Clingfilm basis. Inches are invariably lost, but this comes from losing water and not fat. Meaning, the effect usually lasts for one to two days, and the second you start drinking and eating again, your body will inflate.

Good for little-black-dress moments. Not good for bikini beach days.

Colonic irrigation

This is a 40-minute beauty/health process whereby purified water is pumped through the colon via a tube put up your bottom. Stored faecal matter, gas, mucus and toxic

tip

By the end of three days, you'll hopefully be feeling refreshed and full of vitality. Your skin should glow, your energy levels should be high and your sluggishness a thing of the past. For good health, reintroduce foods slowly and carefully back into your system.

substances then flush their way out of the body. This is said to be the perfect detoxification and stomach flattener for those who are desperate. However, it's not sexy, it's not glam and it's not pleasant if you eat junk, take in zero fibre, dilute your diet with hardly any water and mix it with stress.

Good for detoxification and de-bloating. Not good for anyone who is squeamish.

De-bloat through your diet

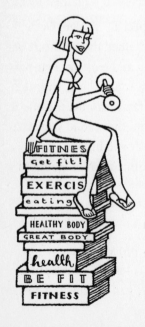

A bloated tummy (think puffed up and as tight as a drum) is usually the result of a poor diet. A diet high in fibre and low in fat and with plenty of water, helps your food pass through your system without strain. If you don't eat healthily, food moves too slowly through your bowel and you will feel bloated. Always choose foods that are naturally high in fibre – wholegrain cereals, granary breads, porridge, fruits, green, leafy vegetables, and nuts and salad – cut back on processed, fatty foods. Next, drink more water; contrary to popular opinion this won't leave you feeling full, but leave your tummy feeling flat.

Find your food intolerance

This is especially important if you have pain after eating and if you have bloating and wind. A study from Addenbrooke Hospital, Cambridge, found that the avoidance of certain foods helped two-thirds of patients with erratic bowel habits. Wheat was reported to be the most common food for aggravating the bowel.

Bash your cellulite

It resembles dimply orange peel, appears mainly on the thighs and bottom and affects 85 per cent of us. The good news is you can beat it and without paying out for expensive creams or downing gallons of water. Cellulite is just body fat, and its appearance is all down to a lack of the male hormone testosterone. It's this hormone that strengthens the fibres of the skin (collagen), which in turn helps hold fat cells together (think about it – fat men don't get cellulite because they still have ample amounts of testosterone in their body to hold their fat cells together). Without it things literally collapse in the presence of body fat, which is why cellulite appears. The good news is you can beat it by:

> **tip**
>
> Don't waste your money on expensive anti-cellulite creams.

1 Eating the right foods:

Reducing the level of fat in the blood is key. Aim for foods rich in omega 3 essential fatty acids (EFAs). These not only regulate the speed at which fat is released into the body but also research shows that they have a definite anti-cellulite effect. EFAs are found in oily fish, especially salmon, and tuna, flaxseeds, linseeds and nuts. Ensure you eat oily fish at least twice a week or take a supplement.

2 Upping your intake of antioxidants:

These help eradicate free radicals – naturally occurring rogue molecules – which also damage the shape of fat cells. Antioxidants can be found in onions, cloves and garlic and Vitamins A, C and E, plus the minerals selenium, zinc and manganese.

3 Exercise:

The number-one way to beat it – see Chapters 3, 4, 5 and 6.

Cellulite isn't cured by:

- Vigorous skin brushing.
- Cutting out caffeine and smoking (though these aren't the healthiest habits even for a lazy girl).
- Expensive creams.
- Massages.
- Body wraps.

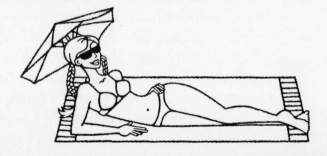

Adapt your everyday eating habits

Let's be honest, if you're reading this chapter you're not going to stop going out to eat, which means it pays to know what the healthy options are in less than healthy food pit stops.

Your local Indian

Unhealthy: a chicken korma, naan bread and pilau rice have 91g (3¼oz) of fat and 1,700 calories.

Healthier: tandoori chicken and plain rice have 35g (1¼oz) fat and 600 calories.

Avoid: creamy curries, anything with coconut, the paneer cheese dishes, fried dishes and poppadums.

Opt for: tandoori or tikka chicken/fish dishes, as these are oven-baked and very low in fat. Pick plain rice over the fancier rice dishes, and vegetables without a heavy sauce.

The kebab place

Unhealthy: doner kebab and chips have 52g (2oz) of fat and 1,135 calories.

Healthier: chicken kebab and salad have 30g (1oz) of fat and 600 calories.

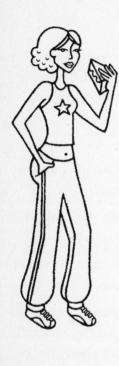

Avoid: the doner kebab – it's loaded with fat, and say no to chips and burgers.

Opt for: a chicken kebab – it's grilled and low in fat, and opt for salad with no dressing.

Pizza

Unhealthy: pepperoni pizza with garlic bread have 65g (2¼oz) of fat and 1,800 calories.

Healthier: cheese and tomato pizza with extra vegetables have 26g (1oz) of fat and 1,100 calories.

Avoid: thin crust, twisted crust, cheese crust – these are all heaped with extra fat.

Opt for: thick crust (or thin, if wood-oven baked), ask for less cheese and top up on toppings like vegetables, egg, fish and chicken.

Chinese food

Unhealthy: sweet-and-sour chicken, egg-fried rice and a spring roll have 72g (2¼oz) of fat and 1,500 calories.

Healthier: chicken stir-fries or prawns in a ginger sauce with plain rice have 21g (¾oz) of fat and 600 calories.

Avoid: egg-fried rice, spring rolls, fried noodles, crispy beef and crispy duck – these are all steeped in fat.

Opt for: Plain rice, boiled vermicelli rice noodles, stir-fried chicken and fish dishes, and vegetables.

Burgers

Unhealthy: cheeseburger with fries and onion rings with coke have 74g (3oz) of fat and 1,400 calories.

Healthier: plain hamburger and small fries with diet coke have 25g (1oz) of fat and 500 calories.

Avoid: the triple, double whammies with cheese, mayo and extra fries with a milkshake.

Opt for: smaller sized hamburger without mayo and cheese, but have two and delete the extra fries.

Fish and chips

Unhealthy: fried cod and chips have 44g (1½oz) of fat and 1,000 calories.

Healthier: ask for a half portion, as it will be just as filling, and it has 22g (¾oz) of fat and 500 calories.

Avoid: large portions of fish, the extra sausage, meat pies and extra chips.

Opt for: smaller portions of everything, and a diet drink.

Fried chicken

Unhealthy: three pieces of chicken, chips and coleslaw have 60g (2oz) of fat and 1,000 calories.

Healthier: skinless chicken burger and baked beans with a diet cola have 13g (½oz) of fat and 490 calories.

Avoid: bargain buckets of fried chicken. With fried chicken half the calories come from fat; also avoid chicken bites, which have little meat, and are heavy in fat.

Opt for: skinless chicken breasts, which are leaner and have less fat. Avoid coleslaw, which is loaded with mayo.

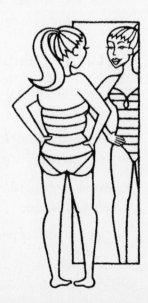

20 lazy ways to get more exercise in your life

1 Make the bed every day

Taking off sheets, turning the mattress, pulling sheets straight, tucking sheets in, plumping up pillows and duvets can burn off at least 50–100 calories.

2 Use your time effectively

Do lunges while watching TV: step forward with one leg, and then drop the knee behind to the floor – keep both knees directly over the feet and drop your bottom towards the floor. This will work your leg and bottom muscles. Combine it with squats (see Chapter 4) and you'll burn 100 calories.

3 Dig up your garden once a week

Or mow your dad's lawn. That will use up 150–350 calories in an hour.

4 Run for the bus every day

A five-minute sprint burns around 100 calories.

5 Do more housework

Vacuuming, ironing, dusting and hanging out washing can all burn an extra 100 calories.

6 Have more sex

Thirty minutes of sex in the morning at a fairly active pace is worth an hour in the afternoon in terms of boosting your metabolic rate and burning fat. Calories used: 250 per 30-minute session.

7 Shimmy in the shower

Do some calf raises (go up on your toes holding for one second and then going go down and repeat 10 times) this will work your calf muscles and bottom.

8 Crunch during bath time

Lie face up on the floor with your feet on the edge of the bath and do three sets of 12 stomach crunches as your bath fills up.

9 Exercise while you cook

Do 20 press-ups against the wall. Muscles used: back, triceps, chest and shoulders.

10 Work at your desk
Sit up straight with your feet on the ground and pull your belly button to your spine and hold it there for 20 counts, release and repeat ten times.

11 Squeeze your bum at the bus stop
Clench and squeeze your bottom cheeks together really hard for ten seconds, five times a day and you'll notice a difference in two weeks.

12 Wash your car
Do it every week and you'll burn 316 calories.

13 Go grocery shopping (and we're talking a big shop)
Then carry it home and you'll burn 246 calories.

14 Vigorously towel off after a shower
And you'll burn 50 calories. Start with a pre-shower body-brushing session and you'll double up to 100 calories.

15 Paint your bedroom
Give it two coats and you'll burn 300–600 calories.

16 Run upstairs for five minutes
Sorry it only counts when you're going up – and you'll burn 100 calories.

17 Skip with a rope
You'll burn 250 calories in ten minutes.

18 Go back to childhood
Invest in some roller blades and, to go faster, bend your knees and push your feet out to the sides. You'll burn 300 calories in 15 minutes.

19 Fidget all the time
Studies show people who can't keep still burn off more calories than those who are naturally more contained.

20 Stop comparing your body to everyone else's
It will help you to feel happier, look fabulous and generally be the most gorgeous person in the room.

chapter 8

How to be extremely knowledgeable about diet and fitness (*without trying*)

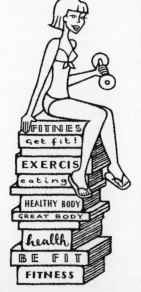

Abdominals

Technical version: this is the band of muscle that traditionally makes up the 'six pack' stomach look.

Lazy girl's version: the part of your stomach that shouldn't roll up when you sit down.

Essential for: a flat stomach and a strong back

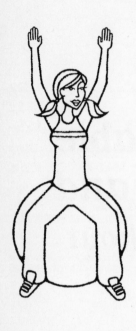

Aerobic exercise

Technical version: this is exercise that requires oxygen and so raises the heart rate. It also improves lung capacity and burns fat.

Lazy girl's version: exercise that allows you to run for a bus without turning blue and passing out.

Essential for: a long and healthy life.

Alexander Technique

Technical version: posture technique that teaches you how to sit, stand, bend and use your spine effectively to banish back pain and improve your posture.

Lazy girl's version: the perfect way to learn how to look like a supermodel.

Essential for: people who are too lazy to stand up straight.

Anaerobic

Technical version: exercise that doesn't require oxygen. This usually occurs during fast or hard bursts of exercise, such as weight lifting.

Lazy girl's version: exercise that exhausts you quickly because you're over exerting yourself.

Essential for: fast-impact sports, such as sprinting and squash.

Antioxidants

Technical version: these mop up the damage everyday nasties, such as smoke and pollution, do to your body. Keep levels high and you'll age slower. Antioxidants can be found in brightly coloured vegetables, such as tomatoes, peppers and leafy green vegetables and also in fruits with a high vitamin C content.

Lazy girl's version: your mum wasn't kidding when she said eat your vegetables!

Essential for: cancer-fighting properties and anti-ageing benefits.

Aqua aerobics

Technical version: a powerful and efficient workout, which tones the body and burns around 700 calories in an hour! The benefits include fat burning, a boost to the metabolism, major resistance work and an increase in your heart and lung capacity.

Lazy girl's version: legs, bums and tums underwater.

Essential for: a long, lean and strong body.

Back pain

Technical version: pain usually owing to weak stomach muscles, which means the back muscles have to support both the back and front of the body.

Lazy girl's version: gain better posture and stronger abdominal muscles and you'll never have any pain.

Essential for: showing you that you need to work on your core muscle groups.

Body Mass Index

Technical version: Body Mass Index (BMI), works out your weight in relation to your height, and is regarded by dieticians and doctors as the standard by which to measure body weight. This is because the BMI can tell you how healthy your current shape is, which is essential in terms of your health.

Lazy girl's version: a statistic that tells you how close you are to being a couch potato.

Essential for: knowing if you're fit or fat.

Biceps

Technical version: the muscle at the front of the upper arm.

Lazy girl's version: the little bump that should appear when you bend your elbow.

Essential for: lifting things, and giving you sexy-looking arms.

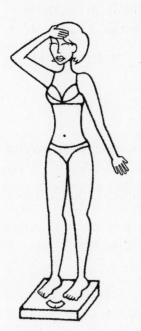

Calories

Technical version: the unit for measuring the energy value of food (so you can work out how much you're taking in, and how much you're burning off).

Lazy girl's version: just one way to tell if you're eating too much (as if you didn't already know).

Essential for: weight loss.

Carbohydrates

Technical version: foods, such as bread, whole grains, pasta and fruit and vegetables, which are used as a fuel source for the body.

Lazy girl's version: food that you should aim to eat five or six portions of each day.

Essential for: energy.

Cellulite

Technical version: deposits of normal fat collected under the skin, leading to a dimpled-dough look.

Lazy girl's version: squishy, orange-peel skin on the thighs and bottom. The result of doing all the things you love to do (lazing about and eating junk food) but know you shouldn't.

Essential for: alerting you to the fact that you need to do some exercise.

Colonic irrigation

Technical version: flushing out the bowel using purified water through the colon via a tube.

Lazy girl's version: a pipe up the bottom to flush out your bottom.

Essential: if you can't get it out any other way.

Detox

Technical version: a spring-clean system where you limit your diet for a short period of time in order to rid the body of harmful toxins that slow your system down.

Lazy girl's version: the diet that eliminates everything you like to eat.

Essential for: brighter skin and weight loss.

Dumbbells

Technical version: a free weight that's designed to be lifted with one hand.

Lazy girl's version: those large, heavy things weightlifters carry around gyms.

Essential for: building lean muscle mass.

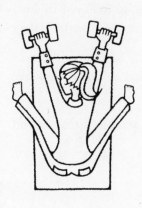

Essential fats

Technical version: omega 3 and 6 fatty acids – the good fats that are vital for the nervous system and the brain.

Lazy girl's version: oily fish – salmon, tuna, mackerel – nuts and seeds, such as pumpkin and flax seeds.

Essential for: glowing skin and a healthy cardiovascular system.

Heart rate

Technical version: the level at which your heart has to pump in order to circulate blood around your body. The harder you exercise, the stronger the heart gets and the more blood it can pump with less effort.

Lazy girl's version: that pounding you hear when you've exerted yourself.

Essential for: staying alive.

Interval training

Technical version: an intense technique where you do short bursts of high-intensity exercise followed by low-intensity exercise (to bring your heart rate down) and then high-intensity exercise again.

Lazy girl's version: a good way to stay awake when you're on the treadmill.

Essential for: building stamina, aerobic strength and burning fat.

Lactic acid

Technical version: a waste product, the result of anaerobic training (lifting weights), which causes muscle fatigue.

Lazy girl's version: the aching pain (not sharp) that you get in your muscle that literally stops you from doing any more repetitions until you've had a rest.

Essential for: helping your muscles to become healthier.

Liposuction

Technical version: a cosmetic-surgery procedure whereby a tube is stuck into a small incision in the skin and fat is literally vacuumed out. Usually used on inner thighs, bottoms, chins and stomachs.

Lazy girl's version: what you'll be doing when you're 50 if you don't get off your backside now.

Essential for: not essential, but one of the most popular cosmetic procedures around.

Low-impact aerobics

Technical version: a workout that raises the heart rate and works the muscles without resorting to high-impact movements, such as running and jumping.

Lazy girl's version: a form of aerobics that's easy on your joints.

Essential for: a healthy heart and toned muscles.

Metabolic rate

Technical version: the rate at which your body burns calories for energy.

Lazy girl's version: how your body uses up that Mars bar you just ate.

Essential for: energy and weight loss.

Olestra

Technical version: a fat substitute used in food (noted on labels). Supposedly the next big thing in diet control, it promises you can eat Olestra-coated food and not get fat.

Lazy girl's version: fake fat that doesn't add calories but could give you the stomach runs.

Essential: if you still intend to eat large packets of junk food.

Organic food

Technical version: food that has been grown naturally without the use of pesticides or GM technology.

Lazy girl's version: food that looks grubby and oddly shaped but is natural and, therefore, better for your health (but not your purse).

Essential for: healthy eating.

Osteoporosis

Technical version: brittle-bone disease that affects women who haven't developed a high bone density by the time they are 30 (when you naturally start to lose bone mass). Mainly owing to lack of calcium, a poor diet, smoking, drinking, and basically being a couch potato.

Lazy girl's version: just one more reason to do some exercise.

Essential for: warning you to look after your bones when you're young.

Pilates

Technical version: a mind-body exercise regime that's akin to a very dynamic form of yoga. Based on building the body's core group of muscles, body realignment and resistance work.

Lazy girl's version: famous-person exercise regime.

Essential for: flat stomach and a healthy back.

Personal trainers

Technical version: individuals trained in all areas of fitness in order to help you achieve your exercise goals, whether they be weight loss, increased stamina or training for a particular sports event.

Lazy girl's version: the person you pay to shout at you when you're at the gym!

Essential for: the body of an athlete.

Pronate

Technical version: a term to describe your foot turning outwards when you run/walk.

Lazy girl's version: if your heels are worn down more on the outside than the inside (this is known as supinate), your foot pronates.

Essential when: buying running shoes, as this should be taken into account to make sure that your foot is properly supported.

Protein

Technical version: one of the main building blocks of the body used to make hormones, give you energy and build muscle – meaning you need to eat at least 35g (1¼oz) of protein a day.

Lazy girl's version: eggs, soya, lean meats, fish, cheese, beans and nuts.

Essential for: a strong and healthy body.

Protein-only diets

Technical version: diets that focus on eating protein-only foods in order to kick-start something called ketosis, which is where the body begins breaking down everything to burn calories.

Lazy girl's version: a bad-for-your-health diet, as, apparently, choosing to chow down on bacon, steaks, burgers, eggs and cheese, over potatoes, bread and pasta is bad for your health (as if we didn't know that).

Essential for: no one really.

Refined foods

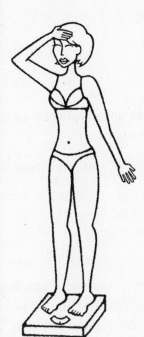

Technical version: foods that are no longer in their 'whole' state, and are pre-packaged usually with added sugars, fats and white flours.

Lazy girl's version: junk food – bad for your waistline and energy levels.

Essential for: fast pick-me-ups but not much else.

Repetitions

Technical version: the number of times you lift and lower a weight in one set, i.e., do three sets of 12 repetitions (that's lift and lower the weight 36 times) before moving to a different exercise.

Lazy girl's version: the number of times you have to do an exercise for it to have an effect on your muscles.

Essential for: building lean muscle mass.

Resistance training

Technical version: working with weights or using your body weight as a force to work against.

Lazy girl's version: all that hard stuff, like squats, and push-ups.

Essential for: a strong, toned body.

Triceps

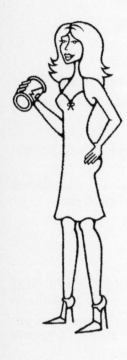

Technical version: the muscle on the underneath of your arm that rarely gets used when lying on the sofa.

Lazy girl's version: the batwing part of your arm (your granny has this).

Essential for: sexy arms.

Vitamins

Technical version: naturally occurring substances, which are essential for a healthy body and life. The best way to get them is through your food intake because this aids their integration into the body and helps them to work effectively.

Lazy girl's version: all the nutrients you avoid if you stick to a low-calorie, or junk-and-alcohol-based diet.

Essential for: fit and healthy bodies.

Yoga

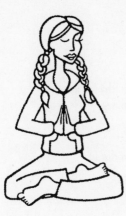

Technical version: ancient Indian body technique designed to promote flexibility, strength and stamina.

Lazy girl's version: bendy, body stuff.

Essential for: a long, lean body.

Yo-yo dieting

Technical version: the process of losing and gaining weight in a repeated cycle.

Lazy girl's version: being a diet junkie.

Essential for: proving to yourself it's not a permanent way to lose weight.

Zzzz... sleep

Technical version: what your body's gagging to do after being up for 16 hours.

Lazy girl's version: something you can actually do without getting off the couch.

Essential for: fabulous looks.

Resources

UK

BackCare – the national association for healthy backs
Tel: 0208 977 5474 Website: www.backpain.org

British Nutrition Foundation
Tel: 0207 404 6504 Website: www.nutrition.org.uk

British Osteopathic Information
Information and advice:
Tel: 01582 488455 Website: www.osteopathy.org

British Wheel of Yoga
Tel: 01529 306851 Website: www.bwy.org.uk

The Colonic International Association
16 Drummond Ride
Herts HP23 5DE
Tel: 01442 827687

Fitness websites
www.thefitclub.com
www.thefitmap.com
www.fitnessheaven.com
www.caloriecounter.co.uk

Gym equipment websites

www.personaltrainer.uk.com
www.weightlosscenter.co.uk
www.yogamad.com
www.totallyfitness.com

Gym websites

Cannons – www.cannons.co.uk
David Lloyd Clubs – www.davidlloydclubs.co.uk
Holmes Place – www.holmesplace.co.uk
LA Fitness – www.lafitness.co.uk

Massage

For a round up of all the massage therapies available in the UK and practitioners in your area go to www.massagetherapy.co.uk

National Centre for Eating Disorders
54 New Road
Esher
Surrey
KT10 9NU
Tel: 01372 469493 Website: www.eating-disorders.org.uk

OUTFIT – Urban Sportswear
32 Middle Lane
Crouch End
London N8 8PL
Tel: 0208 348 6543

Personal trainers

To find your nearest trainer call
National Register of Personal Trainers
Tel: 0870 200 6010 Website: www.nrpt.co.uk
Association of Personal Trainers
PO Box 174
Hastings TN32 5WA
Tel: 01424 465333 Website: www.aopt.co.uk

Pilates

Pilates Off the Square Website: www.pilatesoffthesquare.co.uk
For a trained teacher in your area contact
The Pilates Foundation
Tel: 07071 781859 Website: www.pilatesfoundation.com

Society of Chiropodists
54 Station Road
London NW10 4UA
Tel: 0208 961 4006 Website: www.feetforlife.org

Swiss ball

ProActive Health – Tel: 0870 84 84 842
Totally Fitness – Tel: 0207 467 5925

Walking

Website: www.walking.org

Yoga links

www.bikramyoga.com – Bikram Yoga
www.triyoga.com – Triyoga, London
www.iyi.org.uk – Iyengar yoga

www.bwy.org.uk – British Wheel of Yoga
www.sivananda.org – Sivananda yoga

Australia

www.healthandfitness.com.au – fitness site
www.fitnessaustralia.com.au – fitness tips
www.fitnessonline.com – personal trainers and gyms
www.onlyfitness.com.au – fitness tips and trainers
www.sissel-online.com – Swiss ball and gym equipment
www.pilates.net – Pilates Institute of Australasia
www.iyta.org.au – international yoga teachers

New Zealand

www.everybody.co.nz – health and fitness tips
www.clinicalpilates.com/nz.htm – Pilates
www.yoga.co.nz – yoga

South Africa

www.bodyline.co.za – nutrition
www.fitnesszone.co.za – gyms, fitness tips, stockists, and yoga
and Pilates
www.bodycontrol.co.uk/south.africa.html – Pilates
www.yoga.com – yoga

North America

www.acefitness.org – American Council on Exercise
www.asics.com – ASICS running shoe site

www.crunch.com – Crunch fitness gyms
www.dietiticians.ca – healthy eating site
www.fitter1.com – Swiss ball stockists
www.fitnessusa.com – personal training, gyms, stockists
www.nike.com – Nike site
www.performbetter.com – Swiss ball and gym equipment stockists
www.sissel-shop-canada.com – home gym equipment
www.shape.com – health and fitness tips
www.yogilates.com – yoga and Pilates information
www.yogacentre.com – yoga gear

index